Study Guide to accompany Christensen & Kockrow

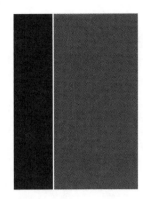

Adult Health Nursing

D0898703

Fourth Edition

Ruth Ann Eckenstein, RN, BS, M.Ed
Program Specialist
Health Occupations Education
Oklahoma Department of Career and Technology Education
Stillwater, Oklahoma

SKILLS PERFORMANCE CHECKLISTS:

Barbara Lauritsen Christensen, RN, MS
Nurse Educator
Mid-Plains Community College
North Platte, Nebraska

Elaine Oden Kockrow, RN, MS
Formerly, Nurse Educator
Mid-Plains Community College
North Platte, Nebraska

MOSBY
An Affiliate of Elsevier

MOSBY, INC.
An Affiliate of Elsevier
11830 Westline Industrial Drive
St. Louis, Missouri 63146

Vice President, Publishing Director: Sally Schrefer
Senior Editor: Terri Wood
Senior Developmental Editor: Robin Richman
Developmental Editor: Catherine Ott
Project Manager: Gayle May

Printed in the United States of America.

International Standard Book Number: 0-323-01753-3

04 05 06 07 08 7 6 5 4 3

Preface

This study guide has been developed as a tool to assist you in evaluating your understanding of the information presented in the *Adult Health Nursing* text. In mastering this information you will be obtaining the knowledge and necessary skills that will be important to you in your nursing practice.

The objectives from each chapter are organized under topic headings. Different learning activities are identified that will assist you to meet the content objectives. This study guide incorporates active learning methods as an educational strategy. *Active learning* is a strategy of engaging the learner in the process of analysis, synthesis, and evaluation of new information instead of being a passive receiver of facts and details. By involving the learner actively and directly, comprehension and retention of knowledge is achieved. This knowledge is easier to remember because it has been organized with learned information already present. Complex relationships among parts or elements are explained as well as clarification of concepts that cannot be communicated easily. Active learning keeps you engaged and involved in making the information yours, assisting you in becoming responsible for acquiring information, and incorporating it into your nursing practice. Active learning activities include matching or defining terms, tables and charts, labeling exercises, chain-of-events, fill-in-the-blanks, and index cards.

Study hints for completion of study guide exercises:

- Read each chapter carefully and highlight or make your own notes or outline of important information.
- Review the **Key Points** presented at the end of each chapter of the *Adult Health Nursing* textbook and complete the study questions.
- Complete the study guide exercises to the best of your ability.
- Page numbers are provided with each learning activity for your reference. Do not look up the correct answers until you have completed a section. You can repeat the exercises if you need to review the information. A complete Answer Key has been provided for your instructor.

In nursing, a strong knowledge base is important, and understanding the basic concepts and principles is necessary in order to be prepared for patient care experiences.

To the Student

This Study Guide was created to assist you in achieving the objectives of each chapter in *Adult Health Nursing*, Fourth Edition, and establishing a solid base of knowledge in medical-surgical nursing. Completing the exercises in each chapter in this guide will help to reinforce the material studied in the textbook and learned in class. Such reinforcement also helps students to be successful on the NCLEX-PN.

Study Hints for All Students

Ask Questions!

There are no stupid questions. If you do not know something or are not sure, you need to find out. Other people may be wondering the same thing but may be too shy to ask. The answer could mean life or death to your patient. That is certainly more important than feeling embarrassed about asking a question.

Chapter Objectives

At the beginning of each chapter in the textbook are objectives that you should have mastered when you finish studying that chapter. Write these objectives in your notebook, leaving a blank space after each. Fill in the answers as you find them while reading the chapter. Review to make sure your answers are correct and complete. Use these answers when you study for tests. This should also be done for separate course objectives that your instructor has listed in your class syllabus.

Key Terms

At the beginning of each chapter in the textbook are key terms that you will encounter as you read the chapter. Text page number references are provided, for easy reference and review, and the key terms are in color the first time they appear in the chapter. Phonetic pronunciations are provided for terms that students might find difficult to pronounce. The terms that were assigned simple phonetic pronunciations were selected because they are either (1) difficult medical, nursing, or scientific terms or (2) other words that may be difficult for students to pronounce. The goal is to help the student reader with limited proficiency in English to develop a greater command of the pronunciation of scientific and nonscientific English terminology. It is hoped that a more general competency in the understanding and use of medical and scientific language may result.

Key Points

Use the Key Points at the end of each chapter in the textbook to help with review for exams.

Reading Hints

When reading each chapter in the textbook, look at the subject headings to learn what each section is about. Read first for the general meaning. Then reread parts you did not understand. It may help to read those parts aloud. Carefully read the information given in each table and study each figure and its caption.

Concepts

While studying, put difficult concepts into your own words to see if you understand them. Check this understanding with another student or the instructor. Write these in your notebook.

Class Notes

When taking lecture notes in class, leave a large margin on the left side of each notebook page and write only on right-hand pages, leaving all left-hand pages blank. Look over your lecture notes soon after each class, while your memory is fresh. Fill in missing words, complete sentences and ideas, and underline key phrases, definitions, and concepts. At the top of each page, write the topic of that page. In the left margin, write the key word for that part of your notes. On the opposite left-hand page, write a summary or outline that combines material from both the textbook and the lecture. These can be your study notes for review.

Study Groups

Form a study group with some other students so you can help one another. Practice speaking and reading aloud. Ask questions about material you are not sure about. Work together to find answers.

References for Improving Study Skills

Good study skills are essential for achieving your goals in nursing. Time management, efficient use of study time, and a consistent approach to studying are all beneficial. There are various study methods for reading a textbook and for taking class notes. Some methods that have proven helpful can be found in *Saunders Student Nurse Planner: A Guide to Success in Nursing School.* This book contains helpful information on test taking and preparing for clinical experiences. It includes an example of a "time map" for planning study time and a blank form that the student can use to formulate a personal time map.

Additional Study Hints for English as a Second Language (ESL) Students

Vocabulary

If you find a nontechnical word you do not know (e.g., *drowsy*), try to guess its meaning from the sentence (e.g., *With electrolyte imbalance, the patient may feel fatigued and drowsy*). If you are not sure of the meaning, or if it seems particularly important, look it up in the dictionary.

Vocabulary Notebook

Keep a small alphabetized notebook or address book in your pocket or purse. Write down new nontechnical words you read or hear along with their meanings and pronunciations. Write each word under its initial letter so you can find it easily, as in a dictionary. For words you do not know or for words that have a different meaning in nursing, write down how they are used and sound. Look up their meanings in a dictionary or ask your instructor or first-language buddy. Then write the different meanings or usages that you have found in your book, including the nursing meaning. Continue to add new words as you discover them. For example:

primary
- of most importance; main: *the primary problem or disease*
- the first one; elementary: *primary school*

secondary
- of less importance; resulting from another problem or disease: *a secondary symptom*
- the second one: *secondary school (in the United States, high school)*

First Language Buddy

ESL students should find a first-language buddy—another student who is a native speaker of English and who is willing to answer questions about word meanings, pronunciations, and culture. Maybe your buddy would like to learn about your language and culture as well. This could help in his or her nursing experience as well.

Contents

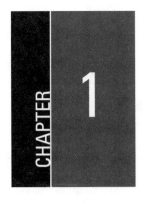

Student Name _____

CHAPTER 1
Introduction to Anatomy and Physiology

Answer Key: Textbook page references are provided as a guide for answering these questions. A complete answer key was provided for your instructor.

MATCHING

Objectives

- Define the key terms as listed.
- Define the difference between anatomy and physiology.

Match the correct definition to the term by placing the letter of the definition next to the term in the "matching letter" column.

		Terms	Matching Letter		Definitions
(8, 9)	1.	Active transport	_____	A.	A group of several different kinds of tissues that perform a special function
(1)	2.	Anatomy	_____	B.	An organization of similar cells that act together
(4)	3.	Cells	_____	C.	The largest organelle within the cell
(5)	4.	Cytoplasm	_____	D.	An organization of varying organs that work together to do complex functions
(10)	5.	Diffusion	_____	E.	A relative constancy in the internal environment of the body
(1)	6.	Dorsal	_____	F.	A substance that exists only in cells
(10)	7.	Filtration	_____	G.	Fundamental unit of all living tissue
(5)	8.	Homeostasis	_____	H.	Type of somatic cell division in which each daughter cell contains the same number of chromosomes as the parent cell
(12)	9.	Membrane	_____	I.	The movement of materials across the membrane of a cell by means of chemical activity

(continued next page)

	Terms	Matching Letter		Definitions
(8)	10. Mitosis	_____	J.	The process that permits a cell to engulf and digest any foreign material
(6)	11. Nucleus	_____	K.	The movement of small molecules across the membrane of a cell by diffusion
(4)	12. Organ	_____	L.	Thin sheets of tissue that serve many functions
(10)	13. Osmosis	_____	M.	The movement of water and particles through a membrane by force from either pressure or gravity
(9, 10)	14. Passive transport	_____	N.	The process by which extracellular fluid is taken into the cell
(9)	15. Phagocytosis	_____	O.	The study, classification, and description of structure and organs of the body
(1)	16. Physiology	_____	P.	To face forward; the front of the body
(9)	17. Pinocytosis	_____	Q.	Explains the processes and functions of the various structures and how they relate to each other
(4)	18. System	_____	R.	The passage of water across a selectively permeable membrane; water moves from less-concentrated solution to more-concentrated solution
(4)	19. Tissue	_____	S.	Toward the back
(1)	20. Ventral	_____	T.	The process in which solid particles in a fluid move from an area of higher concentration to an area of lower concentration

Student Name_____

SENTENCE CONSTRUCTION

Objective

- Use each word of a given list of anatomical terms in a sentence.

Write patient teaching sentences using each term in the exercise above. Be sure that each sentence is written in terms that the patient will understand. (Page references are indicated in exercise above.)

1. _____

2. _____

3. _____

4. _____

5. _____

6. _____

7. _____

8. _____

9. _____

10. _____

11. _____

12. _____

13. _____

14. _____

15. _____

16. _____

17. _____

18. _____

19. _____

20. _____

CELL ART

Objective

- Identify and define three major components of the cell.

Label the parts of the cell. *(6)*

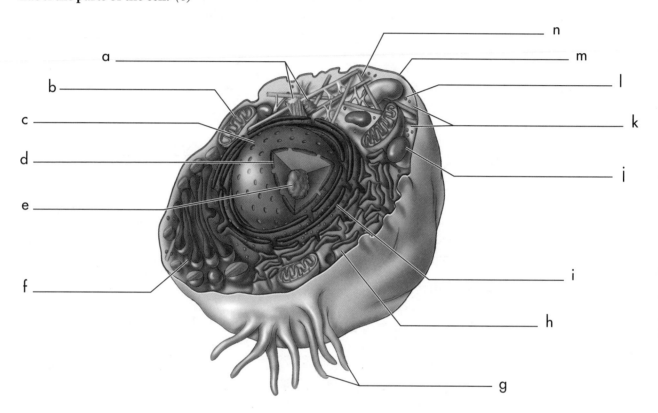

PHASES OF MITOSIS

Objective

- Discuss the stages of mitosis and explain the importance of cellular reproduction.

Next to each phase of mitosis, explain what happens to the chromosomes and the significance of this type of reproduction. *(8)*

Prophase _____

_____

Metaphase _____

_____

Student Name _____

Anaphase _____

_____

Telophase _____

_____

Significance _____

_____

_____

TYPES OF TISSUES

Objective

- Describe the four types of body tissues.

Complete the table below by inserting the types of cells for each group of tissues. *(11-12)*

Epithelial	Connective	Muscle	Nervous
1.	1.	1.	1.
2.	2.	2.	2.
3.	3.	3.	
4.	4.		
	5.		
	6.		

IDENTIFY TYPES OF MEMBRANES

Objective

- Discuss the two types of epithelial membranes.

Identify each type of membrane that is present on the body surface listed in the left column. *(12-13)*

Body Surface	Type of Membrane
Nose	
Lungs	
Intestines	
Bladder	
Mouth	
Vagina	
Heart	
Knee	
Elbow	

MAJOR SYSTEMS—PATIENT OBSERVATION

Objective

- List the eleven major organ systems of the body and briefly describe the major functions of each major organ system.

You are in your patient's room for the first time that morning. List the major systems that you would want to observe, one body part of that system, and why it would be important to make that observation. *(13-15)*

Major System	One Body Part of that System	Importance of Observation
1.		
2.		
3.		

Student Name _____

Major System	One Body Part of that System	Importance of Observation
4.		
5.		
6.		
7.		
8.		
9.		

TYPES OF MUSCLES

Objective

- Describe the four types of body tissues.

Identify the types of muscles and an example of where each type is located. *(13)*

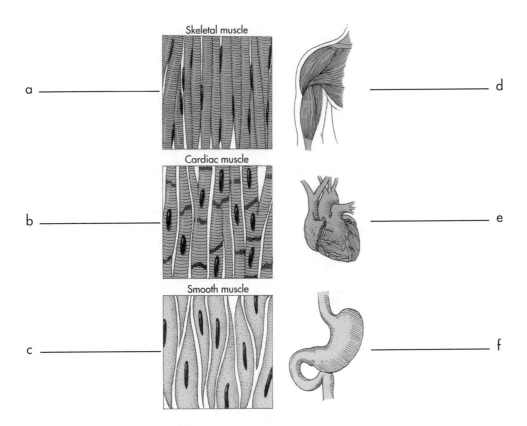

MOVEMENT

Objective

- Differentiate between active and passive transport processes that act to move substances through cell membranes and give two examples of each.

List three types of active and passive transport processes and give two examples of each. *(9, 10)*

Active Transport	Example	Example
1.		
2.		
3.		

Passive Transport	Example	Example
1.		
2.		
3.		

LOCATION OF BODY PARTS

Objectives

- Define the term *anatomical position*.
- List and define the principal directional terms and sections (planes) used in describing the body and the relationship of body parts to one another.

Your patient is standing in front of you in the anatomical position. Next to each body part, label the relationship of that part to the right hand and the head. List the plane where the body part is located. *(2)*

Body Part	Relationship to Right Hand	Relationship to Head	Plane of Body Part
Left hand			
Right foot			
Left shoulder			
Right knee			

Student Name _____

Body Part	Relationship to Right Hand	Relationship to Head	Plane of Body Part
Left elbow			
Chin			
Right pelvic area			
Left posterior buttock			
Right heel			
Left thigh			

FACING THE PATIENT

Objective

- List the nine abdominopelvic regions and the abdominopelvic quadrants.

As you stand at the foot of your supine patient's bed, find the locations of his major organs. Next to each of the nine abdominopelvic regions and the abdominopelvic quadrants, identify a major organ system and one part of that system. *(3, 4)*

Region	Major Organ System	Part of that System
Right hypochondriac		
Epigastric		
Left hypochondriac		
Right lumbar		
Umbilical		
Left lumbar		
Right iliac (inguinal)		
Hypogastric		
Left iliac (inguinal)		

Quadrant	Major Organ System	Part of that System
Right upper		
Left upper		
Right lower		
Left lower		

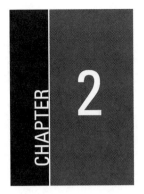

CHAPTER **2**

Care of the Surgical Patient

Answer Key: Textbook page references are provided as a guide for answering these questions. A complete answer key was provided for your instructor.

PATIENT TEACHING USING KEY TERMS

Objective

- Define the key terms as listed.

Develop patient teaching sentences using the following key terms. You may combine more than one term in a sentence and have more than one topic in your patient teaching. Be sure that your patient will understand the meaning of each word.

(20)	Ablation	*(28)*	Infarct
(35)	Anesthesia	*(24-25)*	Informed consent
(44)	Atelectasis	*(20)*	Intraoperative
(44)	Cachexia	*(19)*	Palliative
(48)	Catabolism	*(47)*	Paralytic ileus
(44)	Dehiscence	*(20)*	Perioperative
(41)	Drainage	*(20)*	Postoperative
(28)	Embolus	*(20)*	Preoperative
(44)	Evisceration	*(38)*	Prosthesis
(41)	Extubate	*(48)*	Singultus
(41)	Exudates	*(19)*	Surgery
(26-27)	Incentive spirometry	*(40)*	Surgical asepsis
(31-32)	Incision	*(28)*	Thrombus

_____

_____

_____

_____

_____

_____

_____

_____

_____

_____

_____

_____

_____

_____

_____

_____

_____

_____

_____

_____

_____

_____

_____

_____

_____

_____

_____

_____

_____

Student Name _____

TRUE/FALSE

Objective

- Identify the purposes of surgery.

Determine whether each statement below is true or false. *(20)*

_____ 1. The restoration of function to a lacerated arm is called constructive surgery.

_____ 2. Removal of the appendix is an ablative type of surgery.

_____ 3. A breast biopsy is a palliative surgery.

_____ 4. A diagnostic surgery allows the physician to confirm a diagnosis.

_____ 5. A colostomy usually will not produce a cure.

_____ 6. Total hip replacement is a type of transplant surgery.

_____ 7. Closure of an atrial septal defect in the heart is a constructive surgery.

_____ 8. Internal fixation of a right fibula is reconstructive surgery.

_____ 9. Removal of a mole that has an abnormal appearance is reconstructive surgery.

_____ 10. An ablative surgery is a removal of diseased body part.

SURGERY URGENCY

Objective

- Distinguish between elective, urgent, and emergency surgery.

Explain the urgency of the following types of surgeries. *(20)*

1. Elective _____

_____

2. Emergency _____

_____

3. Urgent _____

_____

TOLERANCE FACTORS

Objective

- Discuss the factors that influence an individual's ability to tolerate surgery.

Each of the following will also affect how a patient will tolerate surgery. Please list why these factors can make a difference in a patient's reaction to surgery. *(20-23)*

Serious illness

Nutrition

Socioeconomic and cultural needs

Education and experience

TC & DB, LEG EXERCISES

Objective

- Explain the procedure for turning, deep breathing, coughing, and leg exercises for postoperative patients.

Develop an index card that will prompt you during your patient teaching for turning, deep breathing, coughing, and leg exercises. Include major steps and enough information to remind you about what to teach your patient. *(23)*

Student Name _____

THE SIGNATURE

Objective

- Explain the importance of informed consent for surgery.

Fill in the blanks below about the importance of the informed consent for surgery. *(24-25)*

Surgical Permit

In signing the informed consent, _____ stated

on the form.

Information is _____ risks

_____, expected benefits _____, and conse-

quences _____.

Witnesses _____

_____.

A witness only _____

_____ consent.

The witness is not _____

_____.

Informed consent should not _____

_____.

Date _____

Patient _____

NURSE'S RESPONSIBILITIES

Objective

- Describe the role of the circulating nurse and the scrub nurse during surgery.

Next to each task indicate with a "C" if it is the circulating nurse's duty, an "S" if it is the scrub nurse's duty, or "CS" if it is both nurses' responsibility. *(38-40)*

Duty	Nurse
1. Performs surgical hand scrub.	_____
2. Performs and confirms patient assessment.	_____
3. Counts sponges, needles, and instruments.	_____
4. Gowns and gloves surgeons.	_____
5. Provides supplies as needed.	_____
6. Assists by tying gowns.	_____
7. Checks medical record for completeness.	_____
8. Documents operative records and nurse's notes.	_____
9. Checks instruments for proper functioning.	_____
10. Assists with surgical draping of patient.	_____
11. Identifies and handles surgical specimens.	_____
12. Observes progress of surgical procedure.	_____
13. Observes sterile field closely for any breaks in aseptic techniques and reports accordingly.	_____
14. Sends for patient at proper time.	_____
15. Transfers patient to gurney for transport to recovery.	_____
16. Maintains neat and orderly sterile field.	_____
17. Prepares operating room with necessary equipment and supplies and ensures that equipment is functional.	_____

Student Name _____

PREOPERATIVE INFORMATION

Objective

- Discuss the preoperative checklist.

List the 21 parts of the preoperative assessment form. Include why it is important to have information regarding each part. *(39)*

Part	Importance
1.	
2.	
3.	
4.	
5.	
6.	
7.	
8.	
9.	
10.	
11.	
12.	
13.	
14.	
15.	
16.	
17.	
18.	
19.	
20.	
21.	

ORAL AIRWAY

Objective

- Describe the role of the circulating nurse and the scrub nurse during surgery.

Label the parts of the airway when the oral airway has been inserted. *(36)*

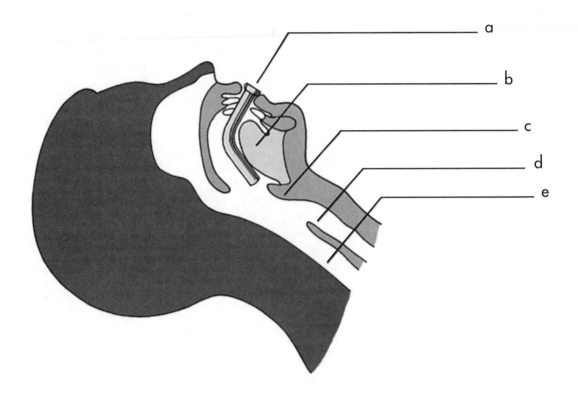

a

b

c

d

e

POSTOPERATIVE CARE

Objective

- Discuss the initial nursing assessment and management immediately after transfer from the postanesthesia care unit.

Your patient has just returned from gastric surgery. Next to each assessment, list what normal findings you would expect and how frequently you would do data collection.

	Assessment	Normal Findings	Frequency
(42)	Vital signs		
(44)	Incision		
(44)	Ventilation		
(46)	Pain		

Student Name_____

	Assessment	Normal Findings	Frequency
(46)	Urinary function		
(46)	Venous status		
(47)	Activity		
(47)	Gastrointestinal		
(48)	Fluids and electrolytes		

RATIONALE

Objective

- Identify the rationale for nursing interventions designed to prevent postoperative complications.

Your patient has just returned from surgery. List the rationale for each nursing intervention to prevent postoperative complications for this patient.

	Nursing Intervention	Rationale
(42)	Vital signs	
(44)	Incision	
(44)	Ventilation	
(46)	Pain	
(46)	Urinary function	
(46)	Venous status	
(47)	Activity	
(47)	Gastrointestinal	
(48)	Fluids and electrolytes	

NURSING PROCESS

Objective

- Discuss the nursing process as it pertains to the surgical patient.

Next to each phase of the nursing process, indicate specifically how that phase relates to the surgical patient. *(48-49)*

Assessment

Nursing diagnoses

Planning

Implementation

Evaluation

PREPARATION FOR DISCHARGE

Objective

- Identify the information needed by the postoperative patient in preparation for discharge.

Develop an index card that contains the major information included in discharge planning for a surgical patient. *(49-51)*

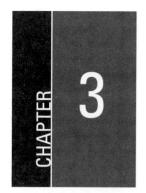
Student Name _____

Care of the Patient with an Integumentary Disorder

Answer Key: Textbook page references are provided as a guide for answering these questions. A complete answer key was provided for your instructor.

STRUCTURES OF THE SKIN

Objectives

- Describe the differences between the epidermis and dermis.

Label the structures of the skin. *(55)*

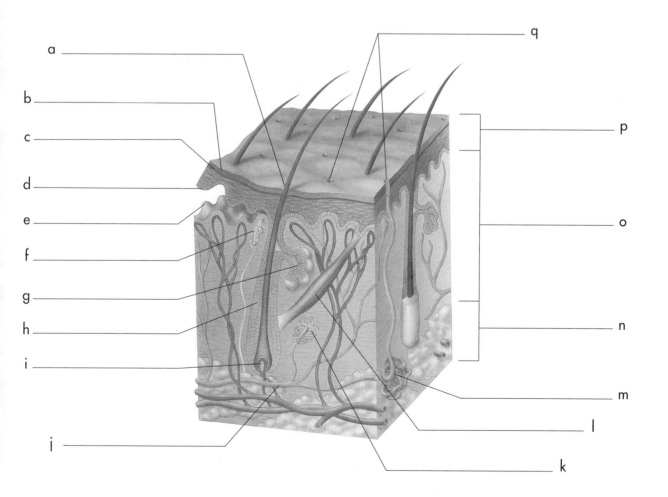

MATCHING

Objectives

Anatomy and Physiology

- Define the key terms as listed.

Medical-Surgical

- Define the key terms as listed.

Match the definition to the terms by placing the letter of the definition in the "matching definition" column provided.

	Term	Matching Definition		Definition
(87)	1. Alopecia	_____	A.	The symptom of itching
(95)	2. Autograft	_____	B.	Circumscribed elevation of skin filled with serous fluid
(92)	3. Contracture	_____	C.	Small, flat blemishes that are flush with the skin surface
(92)	4. Curling's ulcer	_____	D.	Small, raised, solid skin lesions less than 1 cm in diameter
(93)	5. Debridement	_____	E.	Presence of wheals or hives in an allergic reaction
(93)	6. Eschar	_____	F.	Lice infestation; a parasitic disorder of the skin that is usually associated with poor living conditions
(67)	7. Excoriation	_____	G.	Overgrowth of collagenous scar tissue at the site of a wound
(64)	8. Exudate	_____	H.	Round elevation of the skin; white in the center with a pale red periphery
(95)	9. Heterograft (xenograft)	_____	I.	A black, leathery crust (slough) that the body forms over burned tissue that can harbor microorganisms and cause infection
(95)	10. Homograft (allograft)	_____	J.	A benign, viral, warty skin lesion with a rough papillomatous (nipple-like) growth occurring in many forms
(84)	11. Keloids	_____	K.	Removal of damaged tissue and cellular debris from a wound
(70)	12. Macules	_____	L.	Loss of hair
(85)	13. Nevi	_____	M.	Surgical transplantation of any tissue from one part of the body to another

Student Name_____

	Term	Matching Definition		Definition
(73)	14. Papules	_____	N.	Tissue from another species used as a temporary graft
(82)	15. Pediculosis	_____	O.	Small, circumscribed elevation of the skin that contain pus
(57)	16. Pruritus	_____	P.	Transfer of tissue between two genetically dissimilar individuals of the same species
(70)	17. Pustulant vesicles	_____	Q.	Determines the total body surface area (BSA) burned
(89)	18. Rule of Nines	_____	R.	A pigmented, congenital skin blemish that is usually benign but can become cancerous
(71)	19. Suppuration	_____	S.	Shortening or tension of muscles that affects extension
(75)	20. Urticaria	_____	T.	A duodenal ulcer that develops 8–14 days after severe burn on the surface of the body
(84)	21. Verruca	_____	U.	Production of purulent material
(64)	22. Vesicle	_____	V.	Loss of epidermis; linear, hollowed-out, crusted area
(75)	23. Wheals	_____	W.	Fluid, cells, or other substances that have been slowly exuded, or discharged, from small pores or breaks in cell membrane

PROTECTION

Objective

- Discuss the primary functions of the integumentary system.

List the five functions of the skin. *(54-55)*

1. _____

2. _____

3. _____

4. _____

5. _____

LAYERS OF SKIN

Objective

- Describe the differences between the epidermis and dermis.

For each layer of the skin, identify the components for that layer and why they are important. *(55-56)*

Layer	Components	Importance
Epidermis Stratum germinativum		
Stratum corneum		
Melanocyte		
Dermis		
Superficial fascia		

NURSING INTERVENTIONS

Objective

- Identify general nursing interventions for the patient with a skin disorder.

Next to each nursing diagnosis, list nursing interventions that are appropriate for your patient with a skin disorder. *(97-98)*

Nursing Diagnosis	Nursing Interventions
Anxiety related to altered appearance	
Pain related to loss of superficial skin layers	

Student Name_____

Nursing Diagnosis	**Nursing Interventions**

Knowledge deficit related to cause of
skin disorder

Risk for infection related to impaired
skin integrity

Knowledge deficit related to treatment
of skin disorder

Risk for trauma related to symptom
of disorder

Social isolation related to anticipated
or actual response of others to
disfiguring skin disorders

Situational low self-esteem related to
disfiguring skin disorder

NURSING PROCESS

Objective

- Discuss how to use the nursing process in caring for patients with skin disorders.

Next to each phase of the nursing process, indicate specifically how that phase relates to patients with skin disorders. *(96-99)*

Assessment

Nursing diagnoses

Planning

Implementation

Evaluation

PARASITES

Objective

- Identify the parasitic disorders of the skin.

List the parasitic disorders of the skin. *(82-83)*

1. _____

2. _____

Student Name_____

TUMORS

Objective

- Describe the common tumors of the skin.

List the common tumors of the skin and complete the table of information about tumors. *(84)*

Common Tumors

1.   5.

2.   6.

3.   7.

4.

Table of Information About Tumors

Clinical manifestions

Assessment

Diagnostic tests

Medical management

Nursing interventions and patient teaching

DISORDERS OF THE APPENDAGES

Objective

- Identify the disorders associated with the appendages of the skin.

List the disorders of the skin's appendages and the causes of these disorders. *(87)*

1. _____

2. _____

3. _____

4. _____

EXPLANATION OF BURN INJURY

Objective

- State the pathophysiology involved in a burn injury.

Your patient has a severe burn over 20% of her body. She has asked you what will be happening to the area that has been burned. In the space below, explain to her the pathophysiology process that ensues after a burn. She is a science teacher at the local high school. *(87)*

Student Name_____

STAGES OF BURNS

Objective

- Discuss the stages of burn care with appropriate nursing interventions.

List the major nursing interventions for each stage of burn care. *(92)*

Phase	Major Nursing Interventions
Emergent phase	
Acute	
Rehabilitation	

RULE OF NINES

Objective

- Identify the methods used to classify the extent of a burn injury.

Label the body with the Rule of Nines. *(90)*

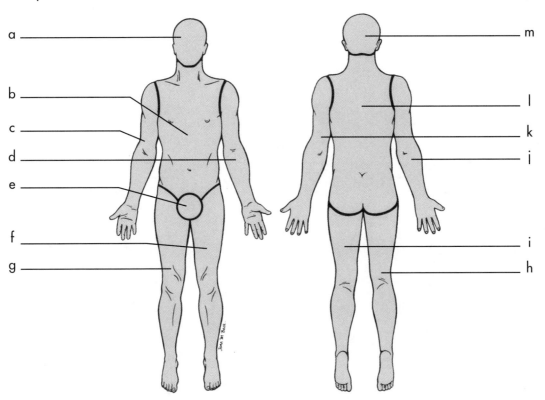

CALCULATE RULE OF NINES

Objective

- Identify the methods used to classify the extent of a burn injury.

Calculate the percentage of burns for each of the situations listed below. *(91)*

1. Nine-year-old child old who was burned while playing with fireworks. She has burns on both of her arms (anterior and posterior), and her anterior chest. _____%

2. A 70-year-old man was burned when he backed up into an open-flame heater. He has burns on the posterior of his body from the ankles to his head. He also has burns on the anterior portion of his legs. _____%

3. Your patient who has diabetes mellitus stepped into a hot shower and has burns on his back and buttocks. _____%

4

Care of the Patient with a Musculoskeletal Disorder

Answer Key: Textbook page references are provided as a guide for answering these questions. A complete answer key was provided for your instructor.

LOCATION OF BONES

Objective

- Describe the location of major bones of the skeleton.

List the bones that are present within each body part. *(103)*

Body Part	Bones
Skull	
Chest	
Abdomen	
Arms	
Legs	
Hands	
Feet	

FUNCTIONS

Objective

- Describe three vital functions muscles perform when they contract.

List three functions muscles perform when they contract. *(103)*

1. _____

2. _____

3. _____

LOCATION OF MUSCLES

Objective

- Describe the location of the major muscles of the body.

Next to the body part, list the major muscles present in that part. *(110-111)*

Body Part	Muscles
Skull	
Chest	
Abdomen	
Arms	
Legs	

Student Name_____

BODY MOVEMENTS

Objective

- List the types of body movements.

Identify the type of movement that each extremity performs when the muscle attached to it contracts.
(106)

Muscles	Extremities	Type of Movement
Pectoralis major	Upper arm	1.
Gluteus maximus	Thigh	2.
Hamstring	Lower leg	3.
Peroneus longus	Foot	4.
Pectoralis major	Upper arm	5.
Tibialis anterior	Foot	6.
Latissimus dorsi	Upper arm	7.
Triceps brachii	Lower arm	8.
Biceps brachii	Lower arm	9.

TERMS

Objectives

- Define the key terms as listed.
- Describe the following conditions: lordosis, scoliosis, and kyphosis.

Define the following terms using medical terminology. In the last column, indicate how you would explain the meaning of that term to a patient.

	Term	Medical Terminology	Patient's Terminology
(118)	Ankylosis		
(112)	Arthrocentesis		

(continued next page)

	Term	**Medical Terminology**	**Patient's Terminology**
(125)	Arthrodesis		
(125)	Arthroplasty		
(131)	Bipolar hip replacement (hemiarthroplasty)		
(165)	Blanching test		
(139)	Callus		
(138)	Colles' fracture		
(143)	Compartment syndrome		
(139)	Crepitus		
(124)	Fibromylagia		
(165)	Kyphosis		
(165)	Lordosis		
(140)	Open reduction with internal fixation (ORIF)		
(158)	Paresthesia		
(165)	Scoliosis		
(124)	Sequestrum		
(157)	Subluxation		
(121)	Tophi		
(144)	Volkmann's contracture		

Student Name_____

DIAGNOSTIC PROCEDURES

Objective

- List diagnostic procedures pertinent to musculoskeletal function.

Explain the following types of diagnostic studies.

(108)   Laminography

(108)   Scanography

(108)   Myelogram

(108)   Nuclear scanning

(109)   Magnetic resonance imaging (MRI)

(109)   Computed axial tomography (CT or CAT scan)

(112)   Bone scan

(112)   Arthroscopy

(112)   Endoscopic spinal microsurgery

(112)   Aspiration

(112)   Arthrocentesis

(112)   Electromyogram (EMG)

DATA COLLECTION

Objective

- Compare methods for assessing circulation, nerve damage, and infection in a patient who has a traumatic insult to the musculoskeletal system.

Your patient has just returned from an application of a long leg cast to her right leg. She fell while hanging wallpaper in her kitchen and broke her right tibia just below her knee. Explain the correct method of determining adequate circulation, possible nerve damage, and infection in her right leg. *(148-149)*

ARTHRITIS

Objective

- Compare the medical regimens for patients suffering from gouty arthritis, rheumatoid arthritis, and osteoarthritis.

List the four goals of medical regimens for patients suffering from gouty arthritis, rheumatoid arthritis, and osteoarthritis. *(113-118)*

1. _____

2. _____

3. _____

4. _____

Student Name_____

NURSING INTERVENTIONS

Objectives

- Discuss the nursing interventions appropriate for rheumatoid arthritis.
- Describe the nursing interventions appropriate for degenerative joint disease (osteoarthritis and ankylosing spondylitis).

Next to each nursing diagnosis, list the nursing interventions that would be appropriate for rheumatoid arthritis, osteoarthritis, and ankylosing spondylitis. *(115-118)*

Nursing Diagnosis	Nursing Interventions
Pain related to joint inflammation	
Pain related to disease process	
Self-esteem, chronic low, related to negative self-evaluation about self or capabilities	
Self-esteem, chronic low, related to body image change	
Knowledge deficit related to lack of information concerning medication and home care management	

LIFESTYLE

Objective

- List at least four healthy lifestyle measures a person can practice to reduce the risk of developing osteoporosis.

List the actions that a woman can take to reduce the risk of developing osteoporosis. *(119)*

1.   5.

2.   6.

3.   7.

4.   8.

SURGERY

Objective

- Describe the surgical intervention for arthritis of the hip and knee.

Your patient has had arthritis of the hip and knee for many years. The medical regimen has failed to relieve the patient's significant pain, resulting in loss of movement. List why surgical intervention would benefit the patient. *(125)*

1. _____

2. _____

3. _____

4. _____

5. _____

Student Name _____

MOVABLE JOINT

Objective

- List the types of body movements.

Label the structures of a freely movable (diarthrotic) joint. *(103)*

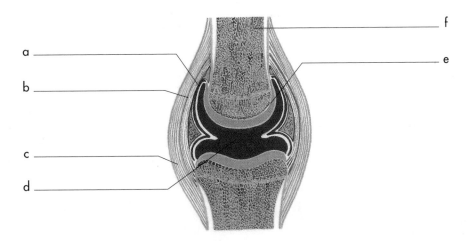

TOTAL HIP OR KNEE REPLACEMENT

Objective

- Describe the nursing interventions for the patient undergoing a total hip or knee replacement.

Your patient has decided to take the doctor's advice and have a total knee replacement. Next to each of the interventions, list the specific nursing actions needed to provide care for your patient after surgery. *(131)*

Positioning

1. _____

2. _____

Wound care

1. _____

2. _____

3. _____

Activity

1. _____

2. _____

3. _____

4. _____

5. _____

6. _____

Pain control

1. _____

2. _____

Discharge instruction

1. _____

2. _____

HIP REPLACEMENT

Objective

- Discuss nursing interventions appropriate for a patient with a fractured hip after ORIF and bipolar hip prosthesis (hemiarthroplasty).

Develop an index card that will prompt you for appropriate nursing interventions for a patient with a fractured hip who has had an ORIF with hemiarthroplasty. *(127)*

FRACTURES

Objective

- Discuss nursing interventions appropriate for a patient with a fractured hip after ORIF and bipolar hip prosthesis (hemiarthroplasty).

Label each type of fracture. *(129)*

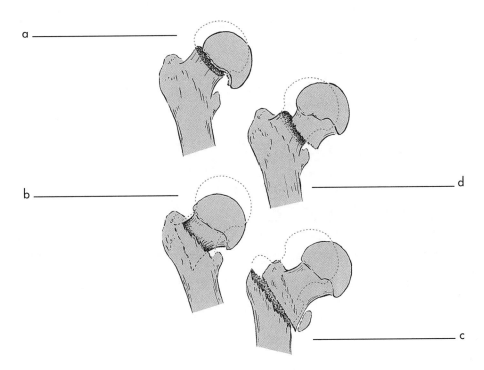

a _____

b _____

_____ d

_____ c

FRACTURE HEALING

Objective

- Discuss the physiology of fracture healing (hematoma, granulation tissue, and callus formation).

Next to each step of fracture healing, explain the physiology of fracture healing. *(139)*

Hematoma

Granulation tissue

Callus formation

COMPARTMENT SYNDROME

Objective

- Describe the signs and symptoms of compartment syndrome.

List the symptoms of compartment syndrome. *(143)*

Subjective

1. _____

2. _____

Objective

1. _____

2. _____

3. _____

4. _____

5. _____

FAT EMBOLISM

Objective

- List nursing interventions appropriate for a fat embolism.

Your patient has been diagnosed with a fat embolism. List appropriate nursing interventions for your patient. *(145)*

1. _____

_____

2. _____

_____

3. _____

_____

4. _____

_____

Student Name_____

TRACTION

Objective

- List at least two types of skin and skeletal traction.

List two types of skin and skeletal traction in the spaces provided. *(150)*

Skin Traction	Skeletal Traction
1.	1.
2.	2.

BONE CANCER

Objective

- List four nursing interventions appropriate for bone cancer.

Your patient has just returned from surgery to remove a large tumor of the left arm. Make an index card of nursing interventions to prompt you during your care of this patient. *(162)*

PHANTOM PAIN

Objective

- Describe the phenomenon of phantom pain.

Explain to your patient why he is complaining of pain in his foot that has been amputatted because of gangrene. *(163)*

CHAPTER 5

Student Name _____

Care of the Patient with a Gastrointestinal Disorder

Answer Key: Textbook page references are provided as a guide for answering these questions. A complete answer key was provided for your instructor.

LOCATION OF DIGESTIVE ORGANS

Objective

- List in sequence each of the component parts or segments of the alimentary canal and identify the accessory organs of digestion.

Label the digestive organs. *(171)*

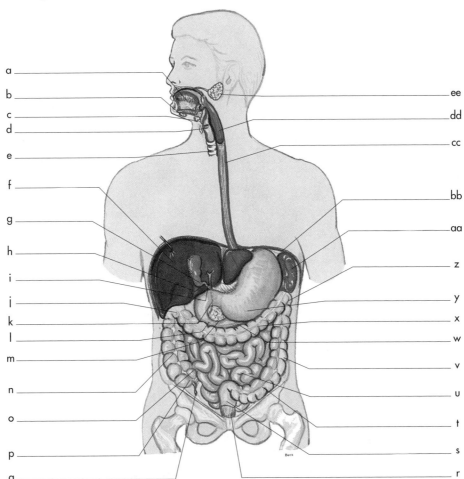

FOOD'S JOURNEY

Objectives

- List in sequence each of the component parts or segments of the alimentary canal and identify the accessory organs of digestion.
- Discuss the function of each digestive and accessory organ.

You have just eaten a piece of cherry pie. List each component part or segment of the alimentary canal and its function as the bite of pie goes down your digestive tract. Be sure to include the accessory organs.

	Component Part	Function
(170)	1.	
(171)	2.	
(171)	3.	
(172)	4.	
(172)	5.	
(173)	6.	
(173)	7.	
(174)	8.	
(174)	9.	

Student Name _____

PATIENT TEACHING USING KEY TERMS

Objective

- Define the key terms as listed.

Develop sentences for a patient teaching presentation using the following key terms. You may combine more than one term in a sentence and have more than one topic in your presentation. Be sure that your patient will understand the meaning of each word.

(182)	Achalasia	*(179)*	Leukoplakia
(175)	Achlorhydria	*(176)*	Lumen
(181)	Anastomosis	*(186)*	Melena
(212)	Cachexia	*(176)*	Occult blood
(212)	Carcinoembryonic antigen (CEA)	*(178)*	Pathognomonic
(194)	Dehiscence	*(198)*	Remission
(182)	Dysphagia	*(202)*	Steatorrhea
(194)	Evisceration	*(201)*	Stoma
(198)	Exacerbation	*(196)*	Tenesmus
(186)	Hematemesis	*(210)*	Volvulus
(177)	Intussusception		

_____

_____

_____

_____

_____

_____

_____

_____

_____

_____

_____

_____

_____

DIAGNOSTIC PROCEDURES

Objective

- Discuss nursing interventions for six diagnostic examinations for patients with disorders of the gastrointestinal tract.

Choose six diagnostic procedures and list nursing interventions that you would use when you are taking care of patients with disorders of the gastrointestinal tract. *(175-178)*

Diagnostic Procedure	Nursing Interventions
1.	
2.	
3.	
4.	
5.	
6.	

Student Name_____

GALLBLADDER AND BILE DUCTS

Objective

- List in sequence each of the component parts or segments of the alimentary canal and identify the accessory organs of digestion.

Label the parts of the gallbladder and bile duct. *(174)*

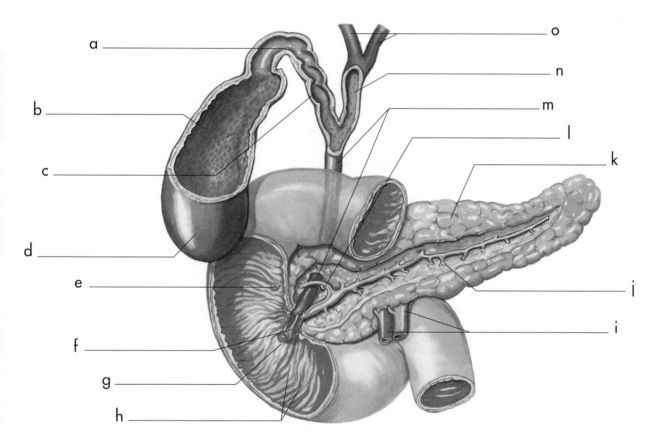

NURSING PROCESS FOR ESOPHAGEAL DISORDERS

Objective

- Use the nursing process to describe nursing interventions for patients with major esophageal disorders.

Next to each phase of the nursing process, indicate specifically how that phase relates to patients with esophageal disorders. *(181-182)*

Assessment

Nursing diagnoses/planning

Implementation

Evaluation

GASTRIC SURGERY

Objective

- Identify nursing interventions for preoperative and postoperative care of the patient who requires gastric surgery.

In the space provided next to each subject, list the nursing interventions that you would take for your patient who is having gastric surgery. *(194-195)*

Preoperative
Preparation
Knowledge
Postoperative
Knowledge
Pain
Noncompliance
Nutrition

Student Name _____

DIFFERENCE

Objective

- Differentiate between irritable bowel syndrome, ulcerative colitis, and Crohn's disease.

List the common etiology, clinical manifestations, diagnostic tests, medical management, and nursing interventions for patients who have irritable bowel syndrome, ulcerative colitis, and Crohn's disease. In the following three columns, list specific information that distinguishes each disorder from the others. *(197-202)*

Common Information

Etiology

Clinical manifestations

Diagnostic tests

Medical management

Nursing interventions

Irritable Bowel Syndrome	Ulcerative Colitis	Crohn's disease

DIVERTICULAR DISEASE

Objective

- Differentiate between diverticulosis and diverticulitis, including medical management and nursing interventions.

List the medical management and nursing interventions for patients with diverticulosis and diverticulitis. *(205)*

Explain the difference between diverticulosis and diverticulitis

Medical management

Nursing interventions

HERNIAS

Objective

- Compare and contrast the types of hernias, including etiology and surgical and nursing interventions.

Under each type of hernia, list the etiology and surgical and nursing interventions for that type of condition. *(208-210)*

	Abdominal	Hiatal
Etiology		
Surgical interventions		
Nursing interventions		

Student Name _____

CANCER

Objective

- Describe the clinical manifestations, surgical procedures, and nursing interventions for the patient with cancer of the colon and rectum.

You are taking care of a patient who has had a bowel resection as a result of cancer of the colon. Develop an index card that will prompt you with information regarding clinical manifestations, surgical procedures, and nursing interventions for your patient. *(211-214)*

FECAL DIVERSION

Objective

- Identify five nursing interventions for the patient with a stoma for fecal diversion.

List five nursing interventions for the patient who has a stoma for fecal diversion. *(213-214)*

1. _____

2. _____

3. _____

4. _____

5. _____

Student Name _____

Care of the Patient with a Gallbladder, Liver, Biliary Tract, or Exocrine Pancreatic Disorder

Answer Key: Textbook page references are provided as a guide for answering these questions. A complete answer key was provided for your instructor.

DEFINITIONS

Objective

- Define the key terms as listed.

Define each of the key terms using terminology that your patient would understand.

(225)   1.   Ascites _____

_____

(229)   2.   Asterixis _____

_____

(227)   3.   Esophageal varices _____

_____

(236)   4.   Flatulence _____

_____

(228)   5.   Hepatic encephalopathy _____

_____

(231)   6.   Hepatitis _____

_____

(232)   7.   Jaundice _____

_____

(243)   8.   Occlusion _____

_____

(227)   9.   Paracentesis _____

_____

(225)   10. Parenchyma _____

_____

(225)   11. Spider telangiectases _____

_____

(236)   12. Steatorrhea _____

_____

NURSING INTERVENTIONS

Objective

- Discuss nursing interventions for the diagnostic examinations of patients with disorders of the gallbladder, liver, biliary tract, and exocrine pancreas.

Next to each of the diagnostic examinations, indicate appropriate nursing interventions for that exam.

	Diagnostic Examination	Nursing Interventions
(221)	Cholecystography	
(224)	Computed tomography of abdomen	
(224)	Endoscopic retrograde cholangiopancreatography	
(222)	Gallbladder scanning	
(223)	Hepatitis virus studies	
(222)	Liver biopsy	
(220)	Liver enzyme	

Student Name _____

	Diagnostic Examination	Nursing Interventions
(222)	Radioisotope liver scanning	
(223)	Serum ammonia	
(223)	Serum amylase	
(220)	Serum bilirubin	
(223)	Serum lipase	
(221)	Serum protein	
(222)	T-tube cholangiography	
(222)	Ultrasound (echogram)	
(224)	Ultrasound of pancreas	
(223)	Urine amylase	

SIGNS AND SYMPTOMS

Objectives

- Define *jaundice* and describe signs and symptoms that may occur with jaundice.
- List the subjective and objective data for the patient with viral hepatitis.

You have a patient with hepatitis. Explain to her what jaundice is and list the objective data that you might observe. *(231-232)*

VIRAL HEPATITIS

Objective

- State the seven types of viral hepatitis, including their modes of transmission.

List the types of hepatitis and how they are transmitted. *(232)*

Type of Viral Hepatitis	Mode of Transmission
1.	
2.	
3.	
4.	
5.	
6.	
7.	

CIRRHOSIS

Objectives

- Explain the etiology, pathophysiology, clinical manifestations, complications, medical management, and nursing interventions for the patient with cirrhosis of the liver.
- Discuss specific teaching content for the patient with cirrhosis of the liver.

List the information on each topic about a patient with cirrhosis of the liver.

(225)   Etiology/pathophysiology

(225)   Clinical manifestations

(226)   Medical management

Student Name_____

(229)   Nursing management

(229)   Patient teaching

ERCP

Objective

- Discuss nursing interventions for the diagnostic examinations of patients with disorders of the gallbladder, liver, biliary tract, and exocrine pancreas.

Label the organs of the body that can be visualized by ERCP. *(224)*

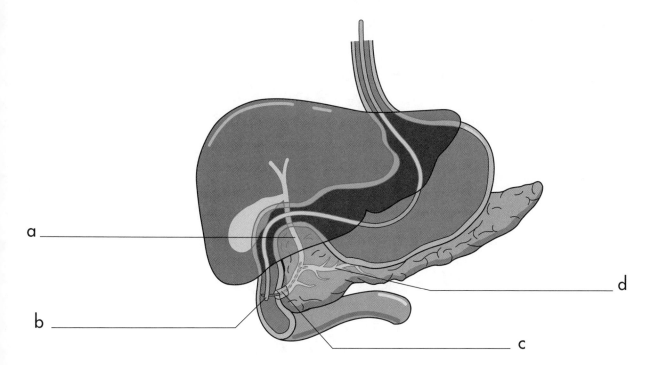

a _____

b _____

c _____

d _____

LIVER, PANCREAS, AND GALLBLADDER

Objectives

- Explain the etiology, pathophysiology, clinical manifestations, medical management, and nursing interventions for the patient with carcinoma of the liver.
- Explain the clinical manifestations, medical management, and nursing interventions for the patient with acute and chronic pancreatitis.
- Explain the clinical manifestations, medical management, and nursing interventions for the patient with carcinoma of the pancreas.
- Explain the etiology, pathophysiology, clinical manifestations, and medical and surgical management for the patient with gallbladder disorders.

Determine the common etiology/pathophysiology, clinical manifestations, medical management, and nursing interventions for carcinoma of the liver and pancreas and acute and chronic pancreatic and gallbladder disease. Then under each disorder list the specific information that differentiates that disorder from the others. Identify the prognosis for each. *(235-247)*

Common

Etiology/pathophysiology

Clinical manifestations

Medical management

Nursing interventions

Student Name _____

Specific Information

Carcinoma of the Liver and Pancreas   Acute and Chronic Pancreatic Disease   Gallbladder Disease

---

COMMON SITES FOR GALLSTONES

Objective

- Explain the etiology, pathophysiology, clinical manifestations, and medical and surgical management for the patient with gallbladder disorders.

Label the common sites for gallstones on this graphic. *(235)*

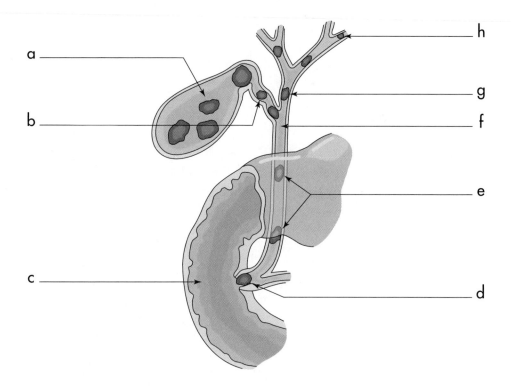

CHAPTER 7

Care of the Patient with a Blood or Lymphatic Disorder

Answer Key: Textbook page references are provided as a guide for answering these questions. A complete answer key was provided for your instructor.

COMPONENTS OF BLOOD

Objectives

- Describe the components of blood.
- Differentiate between the functions of erythrocytes, leukocytes, and thrombocytes.
- Discuss the several factors necessary for the formation of erythrocytes.
- Describe what the *leukocyte differential* means.

Complete the table below with information on the components of blood. *(251-252)*

Component	Common Name	Normal Value	Function	Significance of Abnormality
Erythrocytes				

Factors necessary for the formation of erythrocytes:

Leukocytes—describe what *differential* means.

Component	Common Name	Normal Value	Function	Significance of Abnormality
Neutrophils				

(continued next page)

Component	Common Name	Normal Value	Function	Significance of Abnormality
Eosinophils				
Basophils				
Monocytes				
Thrombocytes				

BLOOD CLOTTING

Objective

- Describe the blood clotting process.

Label each step of the blood clotting mechanism. *(255)*

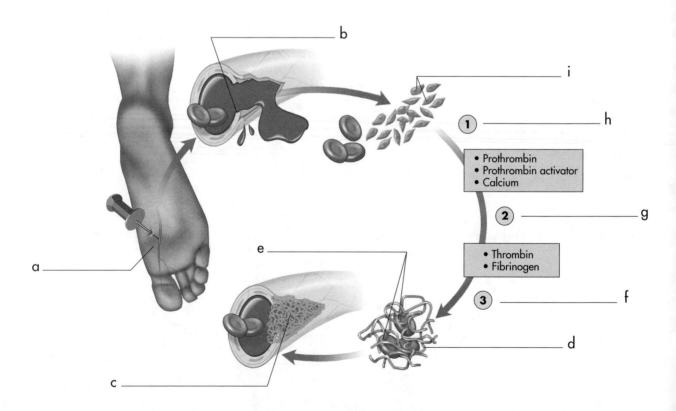

BLOOD GROUPS

Objective

- List the names of the basic blood groups.

List the names of the basic blood groups and which one can be universal donor and which one is the universal recipient. *(254)*

1. _____

2. _____

3. _____

4. _____

ORGANS OF THE LYMPHATIC SYSTEM

Objective

- Describe the generalized function of the lymphatic system and list the primary lymphatic structures.

Label each of the organs of the lymphatic system. *(257)*

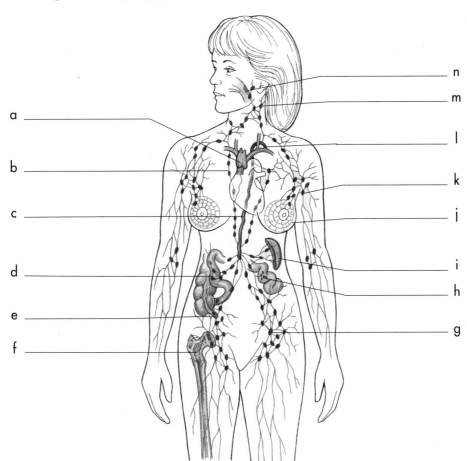

LYMPHATIC SYSTEM

Objective

- Describe the generalized functions of the lymphatic system and list the primary lymphatic structures.

Your patient asked you what the lymphatic system is and why it is important. Explain to her its three functions and next to each structure identify its function. Be sure to explain using terms she can understand. *(255-257)*

Functions

1. _____

2. _____

3. _____

Structures

Lymph and lymph vessels _____

_____

_____

_____

_____

_____

Lymphatic tissues _____

_____

_____

_____

_____

_____

Student Name _____

TERMS

Objective

- Define the key terms as listed.

Match the definition with each term by placing the letter of the definition next to each term.

		Term	Matching Letter		Definition
(258)	1.	Anemia	_____	A.	A hematologic term for a failure of normal process of cell generation and development
(261)	2.	Aplasia	_____	B.	Atypical histocytes consisting of large, abnormal, multinucleated cells in the lymphatic system found in Hodgkin's disease
(274)	3.	Disseminated intravascular coagulation	_____	C.	Causing of great injury and destruction; deadly or fatal
(266)	4.	Erythrocytosis	_____	D.	A malignant disorder of the hematopoietic system in which an excess of leukocytes accumulates in the bone marrow and lymph nodes
(273)	5.	Hemarthrosis	_____	E.	All three major blood elements (RBCs, WBCs, and platelets) from the bone marrow are reduced or absent
(272)	6.	Hemophilia A	_____	F.	A disorder characterized by RBC, hemoglobin, and hematocrit levels below normal range
(264)	7.	Heterozygous	_____	G.	A primary or secondary disorder characterized by the accumulation of lymph in soft tissue and edema
(264)	8.	Homozygous	_____	H.	An inflammation of one or more lymphatic vessels or channels
(271)	9.	Idiopathic	_____	I.	Having two identical genes inherited from each parent for a given hereditary characteristic
(268)	10.	Leukemia	_____	J.	An abnormal decrease in the number of WBCs to fewer than 5000/mm^3
(267)	11.	Leukopenia	_____	K.	A malignant neoplastic immunodeficiency disease of the bone marrow
(277)	12.	Lymphangitis	_____	L.	Having two different genes
(277)	13.	Lymphedema	_____	M.	Antihemophilic factor VIII is absent

(continued next page)

	Term	Matching Letter		Definition
(276)	14. Multiple myeloma	_____	N.	Cause is unknown
(266)	15. Myeloproliferattive	_____	O.	Excessive bone marrow production
(261)	16. Pancytopenic	_____	P.	Bleeding into a joint space
(260)	17. Pernicious	_____	Q.	An abnormal hematological condition in which the number of platelets is reduced to fewer than 100,000/mm³
(279)	18. Reed-Sternberg cell	_____	R.	A grave coagulopathy resulting from the overstimulation of clotting and anticlotting processes in response to disease or injury
(271)	19. Thrombocytopenia	_____	S.	An abnormal increase in the number of circulating RBCs

DIAGNOSTIC TESTS

Objective

- List common diagnostic tests for evaluation of blood and lymph disorders, and discuss the significance of the results.

Explain, by completing the table below, each of the diagnostic tests that is usually done as an evaluation tool for patients with blood or lymphatic disorders. *(257-258)*

Diagnostic Test	Explanation of Procedure	Significance of Results
CBC		
Red cell indices		
Peripheral smear		
Schilling test		
Gastric analysis		
Lymphangiography		
Bone marrow aspiration or biopsy		

Student Name _____

NURSING PROCESS

Objective

- Apply the nursing process to the care of the patient with disorders of the hematological and lymphatic systems.

Develop an index card that highlights the nursing process for patients with disorders of the hematological and lymphatic systems. *(281-282)*

Assessment
Nursing Diagnoses
Planning
Implementation
Evaluation

ANEMIA

Objective

- Compare and contrast the different types of anemia in terms of pathophysiology, assessment, medical management, and nursing interventions.

Next to each type of anemia explain the related pathophysiology, assessment, medical management, and nursing interventions.

Anemia	Pathophysiology	Assessment	Medical Management	Nursing Interventions
(259) Hypovolemic				
(260) Pernicious				

(continued next page)

	Anemia	Pathophysiology	Assessment	Medical Management	Nursing Interventions
(261)	Aplastic				
(263)	Iron-deficiency				
(264)	Sickle cell				

COAGULATION DISORDERS

Objective

- Compare and contrast the disorders of coagulation (thrombocytopenia, hemophilia, DIC) in terms of pathophysiology, assessment, and nursing interventions.

List the common information about thrombocytopenia, hemophilia, and DIC. Then list the information that is specific to each disorder. *(271-276)*

Common Information
Pathophysiology
Assessment
Nursing interventions

Student Name _____

	Thrombocytopenia	Hemophilia	DIC
Pathophysiology			
Assessment			
Nursing interventions			

HEMOPHILIA AND DIC

Objective

- Discuss medical management of patients with hemophilia and DIC.

Your patient wants to know the difference between hemophilia and DIC. Explain the medical management of hemophilia and DIC in terminology that she can understand. *(272-273, 274-275)*

HYPOVOLEMIC SHOCK

Objective

- List six signs and symptoms associated with hypovolemic shock.

You are admitting a patient who has had a traumatic amputation of his right arm. What signs and symptoms of hypovolemic shock could you expect your patient to exhibit? *(260)*

1.

2.

3.

4.

5.

6.

PERNICIOUS ANEMIA

Objective

- Discuss important aspects that should be presented in patient teaching and home care planning for the patient with pernicious anemia.

On the graphic organizer below, list the patient teaching and home care planning for a patient with pernicious anemia. *(260-261)*

	Pernicious Anemia	

PROGNOSIS

Objective

- Discuss the prognoses for patients with acute and chronic leukemia.

You have a patient with chronic leukemia who wants to know the prognosis for her disorder. List the usual prognoses for both acute and chronic leukemia below. *(271)*

Student Name_____

MULTIPLE MYELOMA

Objective

- Discuss the nursing intervention and patient teaching for the patient with multiple myeloma.

Develop an index card that will assist you during nursing interventions and patient teaching for a patient with multiple myeloma. *(277)*

LYMPHEDEMA

Objective

- Discuss the primary goal of nursing interventions for the patient with lymphedema.

List the primary goal of nursing interventions for the patient with lymphedema. *(278)*

HODGKIN'S OR NON-HODGKIN'S DISEASE

Objective

- Differentiate between Hodgkin's disease and non-Hodgkin's lymphomas and related medical management and nursing interventions.

Identify the medical management and nursing interventions for Hodgkin's and non-Hodgkin's lymphomas. *(279-281)*

	Medical Management	Nursing Interventions
Hodgkin's		
Non-Hodgkin's		

CHAPTER 8

Student Name _____

Care of the Patient with a Cardiovascular or a Peripheral Vascular Disorder

Answer Key: Textbook page references are provided as a guide for answering these questions. A complete answer key was provided for your instructor.

TRACING A DROP OF BLOOD

Objectives

- Discuss the location, size, and position of the heart.
- Identify the chambers of the heart.
- List the functions of the chambers of the heart.
- Identify the valves of the heart and their locations.
- Explain what produces the two main heart sounds.

Trace a drop of blood in the aorta backward around the systemic circulatory system ending with the drop of blood back at the aorta: *(290, 291)*

List all of the chambers and valves of the heart and their functions.
Indicate when the blood changes from oxygenated to deoxygenated blood.
Insert the heart sounds and how they are produced.
Name all vessels carrying the blood and what type of blood they carry.

Aorta _____

_____

_____

_____

_____

_____

_____

_____ Aorta

IMPULSE PATTERN

Objective

- Discuss the electrical conduction system that causes the cardiac muscle fibers to contract.

Identify the impulse pattern of the electrical conduction system of the heart, inserting the normal ECG deflections. *(289)*

CORONARY CIRCULATION

Objective

- Trace the path of blood through the coronary circulation.

Label each of the coronary vessels that supply blood to the heart. *(292)*

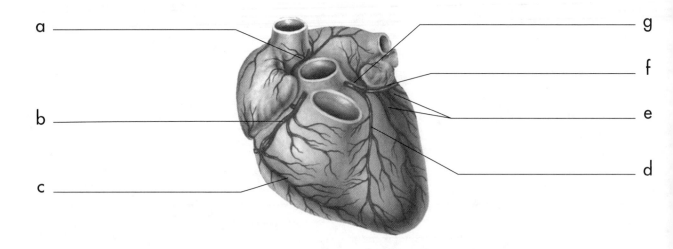

Student Name_____

TERMS

Objective

- Define the key terms as listed.

Define the following using medical terminology. In the last column indicate how you would explain the meaning of that term to a patient.

	Term	Medical Terminology	Patient Terminology
(339)	Aneurysm		
(303)	Angina pectoris		
(332)	Arteriosclerosis		
(332)	Atherosclerosis		
(298)	Bradycardia		
(294)	Cardioversion		
(302)	Coronary artery disease		
(299)	Defibrillation		
(297)	Dysrhythmia		
(308)	Embolus		
(338)	Endarterectomy		

(continued next page)

	Term	Medical Terminology	Patient Terminology
(315)	Heart failure		
(294)	Hypoxemia		
(330)	Intermittent claudication		
(303)	Ischemia		
(308)	Myocardial infarction		
(308)	Occlusion		
(346)	Orthopnea		
(325)	Peripheral		
(316)	Pleural effusion		
(294)	Polycythemia		
(321)	Pulmonary edema		
(297)	Tachycardia		

RISK FACTORS

Objective

- Compare nonmodifiable risk factors in coronary artery disease (CAD) with factors that are modifiable in lifestyle and health management.

Identify which risk factors can be modified and what modification can be taken by the patient to decrease cardiac disease. *(296)*

Risk Factor	Nonmodifiable	Modifiable	Modification by Patients
Smoking	_____	_____	
Age	_____	_____	
Race	_____	_____	
Family history	_____	_____	
Hyperlipidemia	_____	_____	
Diabetes mellitus	_____	_____	
Sex	_____	_____	
Hypertension	_____	_____	
Obesity	_____	_____	
Sedentary lifestyle	_____	_____	
Stress	_____	_____	
Oral contraceptives	_____	_____	
Psychosocial factors	_____	_____	

DIAGNOSTIC TESTS

Objective

- List diagnostic tests used to evaluate cardiovascular function.

Explain the differences among the following types of diagnostic imaging studies.

	Diagnostic Imaging Study
(292)	Fluoroscopy
(292)	Angiogram
(292)	Aortogram
(294)	Thallium 201 scanning
(294)	Echocardiogram
(294)	Positron emission tomogram

You are taking care of a patient who is going to have a cardiac catheterization and angiography studies. Explain the procedures to your patient, including any postprocedure activity restrictions. *(292-293)*

_____

_____

_____

Student Name_____

ABNORMALITIES

Objective

- List diagnostic tests used to evaluate cardiovascular function.

The patient above has had the following diagnostic lab tests. Identify the significance if your patient has abnormal findings for the tests. *(294-295)*

Test	Significance of Abnormalities
CBC	
PT	
ESR	
Na	
K+	
C++	
Mg++	
HDL	
LDL	
ABG	
AST	
CPK/CK	
cTnT	

CARDIAC DYSRHYTHMIAS

Objective

- Describe five cardiac dysrhythmias.

As you enter your patient's room, she asks why markings on the monitor's screen look funny with a lot of high peaks. Explain to her why the monitor is on and what the markings mean. Your patient is in sinus rhythm. *(297)*

_____

_____

_____

Explain the difference in the rate and cause of these dysrhythmias. *(297-299)*

Dysrhythmias	Rate	Causes
Sinus rhythm		
Sinus bradycardia		
Sinus tachycardia		
Supraventricular tachycardia		
Atrial dysrhythmias		
Ventricular dysrhythmias		

PATIENT TEACHING

Objective

- Specify patient teaching for patients with cardiac dysrhythmias, angina pectoris, myocardial infarction, heart failure, and valvular heart disease.

List common patient teaching that you would provide to any patient who has cardiac dysrhythmias, angina pectoris, myocardial infarction, heart failure, or valvular heart disease. *(306-307, 310-313, 319, 323-324)*

_____

_____

Student Name _____

_____

_____

_____

_____

In the table below, add the specific patient teaching that you would provide for your patient with each disorder.

	Disorder	Specific Patient Teaching
(300)	Cardiac dysrhythmias	
(306-307)	Angina pectoris	
(310-313)	Myocardial infarction	
(319)	Heart failure	
(323-324)	Valvular heart disease	

AGING

Objective

- Describe the effects of aging on the peripheral vascular system.

List the changes that occur to the peripheral vascular system as the body ages. *(329)*

Vascular System Part	Changes	Effect of Change
Inner walls		
Middle walls		

NURSING INTERVENTIONS

Objective

- Discuss nursing interventions for arterial and venous disorders.

Place a check next to the nursing intervention that is usually done for patients with arterial or venous disorders. Use the last column to indicate if the intervention can be done for both disorders. *(330-332)*

Nursing Intervention	Arterial Disorders	Venous Disorders	Both
Monitor skin color and temperature	_____	_____	_____
Assess sensation and movement of extremity	_____	_____	_____
Assess peripheral pulses and capillary refill	_____	_____	_____
Monitor extremity for edema	_____	_____	_____
Promote circulation	_____	_____	_____
Avoid sharp flexion of extremities	_____	_____	_____
Administer prescribed NSAIDs	_____	_____	_____
Measure calf or thigh circumference daily	_____	_____	_____
Have patient wear elastic stockings	_____	_____	_____
Avoid crossing the legs at the knee	_____	_____	_____
Elevate legs when sitting	_____	_____	_____
Assess level of discomfort	_____	_____	_____

HYPERTENSION

Objective

- Compare essential (primary) hypertension and secondary hypertension.
- Discuss the importance of patient education for hypertension.

List the common factors between essential (primary) hypertension and secondary hypertension. *(333)*

_____

_____

_____

_____

Student Name_____

Explain why it is important to do patient education regarding hypertension. *(335)*

_____

_____

_____

THROMBOPHLEBITIS

Objective

- Discuss appropriate patient education for thrombophlebitis.

From the list below, check patient education that is appropriate for a patient with thrombophlebitis and explain to the patient the rationale for adherence to the directions. *(343)*

Patient Education	Appropriate	Rationale for Adherence
Maintain diuretic therapy	_____	
Restrict sodium in diet	_____	
Stay in bed in acute phase	_____	
Remove elastic stockings	_____	
Elevate legs when sitting	_____	
Massage extremities when painful	_____	
Avoid flexion-extension exercise	_____	
Avoid crossing legs at knee, tight stockings, or garters	_____	
Encourage ambulation during acute phase	_____	
Monitor calf or thigh circumference daily	_____	

CARDIAC REHABILITATION

Objective

- Discuss the purposes of cardiac rehabilitation.

List the purposes of cardiac rehabilitation. *(315)*

CHAPTER 9

Care of the Patient with a Respiratory Disorder

RESPIRATORY TRACT

Objective

- List and define the parts of the upper and lower respiratory tract.
- Describe the purpose of the respiratory system.

Next to each part of the upper and lower respiratory system, describe the part and list its function. In the last row, describe the purpose of the respiratory system. *(352-354)*

Respiratory Tract Part	Description	Function
Nose		
Pharynx		
Larynx		
Trachea		
Bronchial tree		
Lungs		
Purpose of the Respiratory System		

EXTERNAL/INTERNAL RESPIRATION

Objective

- Differentiate between external and internal respiration.

After your patient's doctor visit, your patient wants to know about internal respiration. Explain the difference between external and internal respiration in terms that your patient will understand. *(351)*

ALVEOLUS AND GAS EXCHANGE

Objective

- List the ways in which oxygen and carbon dioxide are transported in the blood.

Indicate each gas exchange by labeling the places where exchanges occur. *(356)*

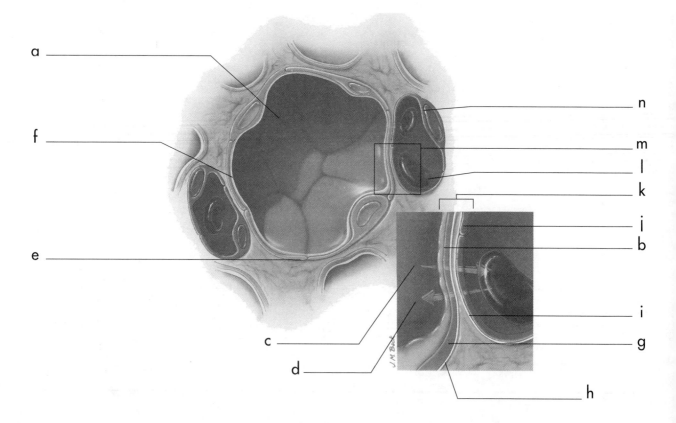

Student Name _____

GAS EXCHANGE

Objective

- List the ways in which oxygen and carbon dioxide are transported in the blood.

Your patient now wants to know how oxygen and carbon dioxide are transported in the blood. Explain how the gases are transported in the blood. *(352)*

REGULATORS

Objective

- Discuss the mechanisms that regulate respirations.

Below the parts of the human body that regulate respiration, explain how the regulation occurs. *(355-357)*

Medulla oblongata and pons of the brain

Chemoreceptors located in the carotid and aortic bodies

TERMS

- Define the key terms as listed.

Define the following using medical terminology. In the last column, indicate how you would explain the meaning of that term to a patient.

	Term	Medical Terminology	Patient's Terminology
(357)	Adventitious		
(386)	Atelectasis		
(359)	Bronchoscopy		
(394)	Cor pulmonale		
(366)	Coryza		
(357)	Crackles		
(364)	Cyanosis		
(357)	Dyspnea		
(391)	Embolism		
(383)	Empyema		
(362)	Epistaxis		
(399)	Exacerbation		
(401)	Extrinsic		
(399)	Hypercapnia		
(386)	Hypoventilation		
(357)	Hypoxia		

Student Name_____

	Term	Medical Terminology	Patient's Terminology
(401)	Intrinsic		
(357)	Orthopnea		
(357)	Pleural friction rub		
(387)	Pneumothorax		
(357)	Sibilant wheeze		
(357)	Sonorous wheeze		
(363)	Stertorous		
(386)	Tachypnea		
(359)	Thoracentesis		
(374)	Virulent		

NURSING INTERVENTIONS

Objective

- List five nursing interventions to assist patients with retained pulmonary secretions.

Your patient is having problems with retaining pulmonary secretions. List five nursing interventions that you can initiate to assist your patient to expel secretions. *(386)*

1. _____

2. _____

3. _____

4. _____

5. _____

INFECTIONS

Objective

- Identify four strategies the nurse can teach patients to decrease the risk of infection.

Develop an index card of four strategies the nurse can teach patients to decrease the risk of infections. *(367)*

ASTHMA OR EMPHYSEMA

Objectives

- Differentiate between medical management of the patient with emphysema and the patient with asthma.
- Discuss why low-flow oxygen is required for patients with emphysema.

List the medical management for a patient with emphysema and asthma. Include why low-flow oxygen is required for patient with emphysema. *(394-399, 401-403)*

Medical Management

Emphysema

Asthma

Rationale for Low-Flow Oxygen for Patients with Emphysema

Student Name _____

COPD OR PNEUMONIA

Objective

- Compare/contrast nursing assessment and interventions for the patient with chronic obstructive pulmonary disease (COPD) and the patient with pneumonia.

In the middle column, list the common assessments and interventions for patients who have COPD and patients with pneumonia. In the left column, insert assessments and interventions for a patient with COPD, and on the right list assessments and interventions for a patient with pneumonia. *(379-382, 394-399)*

Assessments and Interventions for COPD	Common Assessments and Interventions for COPD and Pneumonia	Assessments and Interventions for Pneumonia

DISORDERS OF THE AIRWAYS

Objective

- Differentiate between medical management of the patient with emphysema and the patient with asthma.

Label each disorder. *(395)*

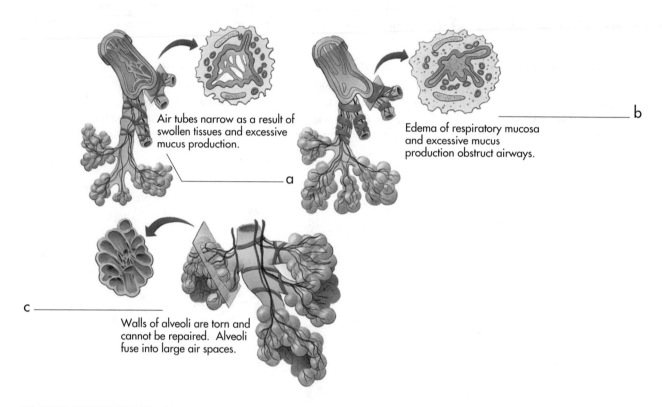

Air tubes narrow as a result of swollen tissues and excessive mucus production.

a

Edema of respiratory mucosa and excessive mucus production obstruct airways.

b

c

Walls of alveoli are torn and cannot be repaired. Alveoli fuse into large air spaces.

CLOSED CHEST DRAINAGE

Objective

- List three nursing assessments/interventions pertaining to the care of the patient with closed chest drainage.

Your have arrived on the nursing unit and found that your patient has been diagnosed with empyema and a closed chest drainage system has been inserted. Listed three nursing assessments and interventions that pertain to the care of the your patient. *(384)*

Nursing Assessments	Nursing Interventions
1.	
2.	
3.	

Student Name_____

LARYNGECTOMY

Objective

- Discuss nursing interventions for the patient with a laryngectomy.

List the nursing interventions for a patient with a laryngectomy. *(366)*

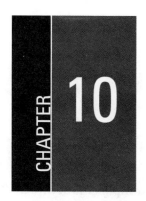

CHAPTER 10

Care of the Patient with a Urinary Disorder

Answer Key: Textbook page references are provided as a guide for answering these questions. A complete answer key was provided for your instructor.

STRUCTURES

Objective

- Describe the structures of the urinary system including functions.

Next to each structure explain its function. *(408-411)*

Structure	Function
Kidneys	
Renal capsule	
Medulla	
Pyramids	
Renal pelvis	
Nephron	
Glomeruli	
Bowman's capsule	
Renal tubule	
Juxtaglomerular apparatus	

URINE

Objectives

- List the three processes involved in urine formation.
- Compare the normal components of urine to the abnormal components.

List the three phases of urine production and then compare normal with abnormal components of urine. *(410-412)*

Three Phases
1.
2.
3.

Comparison of Normal with Abnormal Components of Urine

RENAL TUBULES

Objective

- Describe the structures of the urinary system including functions.

Label each part of the renal tubule. *(410)*

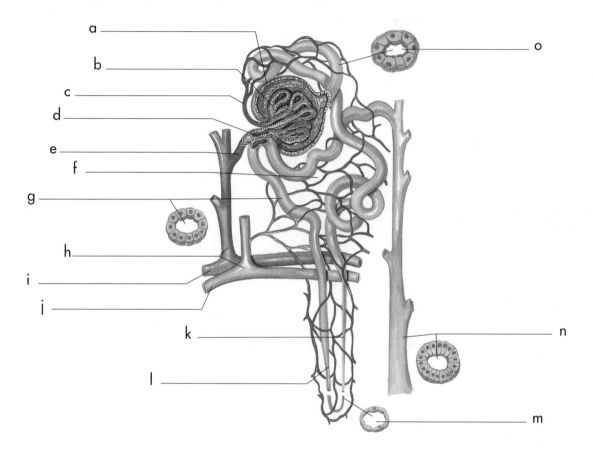

a
b
c
d
e
f
g
h
i
j
k
l
m
n
o

HORMONES

Objective

- Name three hormones and their influence on nephron function.

List the three hormones and their influence on nephron function. *(411)*

Hormones	Influence
1.	
2.	
3.	

TERMS

Objective

- Define the key terms as listed.

Develop sentences for a patient teaching presentation using the following key terms. You may combine more than one term in a sentence and have more than one topic in your presentation. Be sure that your patient will understand the meaning of each word.

(436)	Anasarca	*(447)*	Ileal conduit
(440)	Anuria	*(428)*	Micturition
(424)	Asthenia	*(448)*	Nephrotoxin
(426)	Azotemia	*(424)*	Nocturia
(423)	Bacteriuria	*(436)*	Oliguria
(426)	Costovertebral angle	*(425)*	Prostatodynia
(431)	Cytological evaluation	*(424)*	Pyuria
(443)	Dialysis	*(422)*	Residual urine
(415)	Dysuria	*(421)*	Retention
(424)	Hematuria	*(428)*	Urolithiasis
(427)	Hydronephrosis		

_____

_____

_____

_____

_____

_____

_____

_____

_____

_____

_____

_____

Student Name_____

_____

_____

_____

_____

_____

_____

_____

_____

ALTERATIONS

Objective

- Describe the alterations in renal function associated with disorders of the urinary tract.

Next to each disorder of the urinary tract, list the alterations in renal function.

	Disorder	Alteration in Renal Function
(421)	Urinary retention	
(422)	Urinary incontinence	
(422)	Neurogenic bladder	
(423)	Urinary tract infection	
(424)	Ureteritis	
(425)	Cystitis	
(425)	Prostatitis	
(426)	Pyelonephritis	
(427)	Urinary obstruction	
(427)	Hydronephrosis	
(428)	Urolithiasis	

(continued next page)

	Disorder	Alteration in Renal Function
(430)	Renal tumors	
(430)	Renal cysts	
(431)	Tumors of the urinary bladder	
(431)	Benign prostatic hypertrophy	
(433)	Cancer of the prostate	
(435)	Urethral strictures	
(435)	Urinary tract trauma	
(436)	Nephrotic syndrome	
(436)	Nephritis	
(437)	Chronic glomerulonephritis	
(439)	Acute renal failure	
(440)	Chronic renal failure	

NURSING DIAGNOSES

Objective

- Select nursing diagnoses related to alteration in urinary function.

List nursing diagnoses that relate to alteration in urinary function. *(448)*

1. _____

2. _____

3. _____

4. _____

5. _____

6. _____

7. _____

8. _____

Student Name _____

SPECIAL NEEDS

Objective

- Prioritize the special needs of the patient with urinary dysfunction.

List three special needs of the patient with urinary dysfunction. *(448)*

1.

2.

3.

BODY IMAGE

Objective

- Appraise the changes in body image created when the patient experiences an alteration in urinary function.

Your patient had an ileal conduit inserted 3 days ago because of cancer of the bladder. List appropriate assessments that you would do to determine if she is having body image changes. *(447)*

KOCK POUCH

Objective

- Prioritize the special needs of the patient with urinary dysfunction

Label each part of the Kock pouch. *(448)*

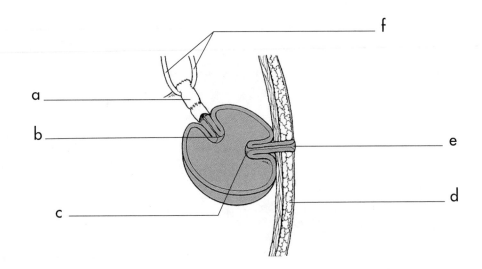

AGING

Objective

- Identify the effects of aging on urinary system function.

List eight effects of aging on the urinary system function. *(413)*

1.   5.

2.   6.

3.   7.

4.   8.

Student Name _____

PATIENT TEACHING

Objective

- Adapt teaching methods for the patient with urinary disorders.

List specific teaching methods for the patient with urinary disorders. *(448)*

Specific Teaching Methods

IMPACT

Objective

- Discuss the impact of renal disease on family function.

List the effects of renal disease on family function. *(440, 442, 445)*

DRUGS AND NUTRITION

Objective

- Incorporate pharmacotherapeutic and nutritional considerations into the nursing care plan of the patient with a urinary disorder.

Develop an index card that would assist you to incorporate pharmacotherapeutic and nutritional considerations into the nursing care plan of your patient with a urinary disorder. *(418-419)*

Student Name _____

CHAPTER 11

Care of the Patient with an Endocrine Disorder

Answer Key: Textbook page references are provided as a guide for answering these questions. A complete answer key was provided for your instructor.

GLANDS AND HORMONES

Objective

- List and describe the endocrine glands and their hormones.
- Explain the action of the hormones on their target organs.

Complete the table below by listing the hormones that each gland produces and the action on their target organs. *(452-456)*

Endocrine Gland	Hormone	Action on Target Organ
Anterior pituitary	1.	
	2.	
	3.	
	4.	
	5.	
	6.	
Posterior pituitary	1.	
	2.	

(continued next page)

Endocrine Gland	Hormone	Action on Target Organ
Thyroid	1.	
	2.	
	3.	
Parathyroid	1.	
Adrenal cortex	1.	
	2.	
	3.	
Adrenal medulla	1.	
	2.	
Pancreas	1.	
	2.	
Ovaries	1.	
	2.	
Testes	1.	
Thymus	1.	
Pineal	1.	

PITUITARY HORMONES

Objective

- List and describe the endocrine glands and their hormones.

Label each gland and identify what hormone it secretes. *(452)*

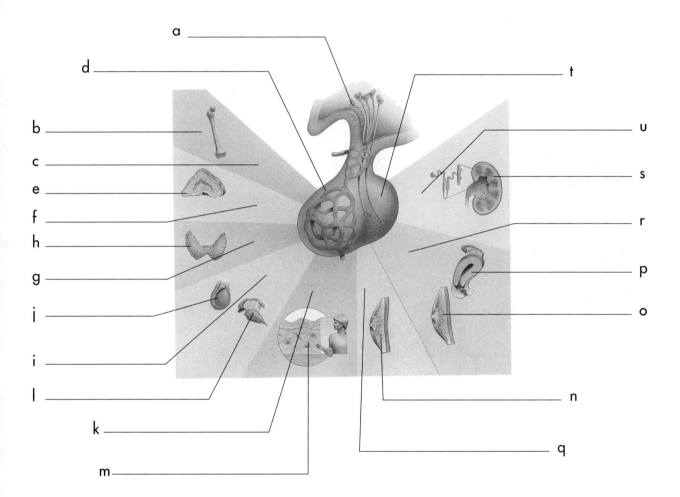

NEGATIVE FEEDBACK

Objective

- Define the negative feedback system.

Prepare a patient teaching presentation on the lines below about the negative feedback system. *(452)*

_____

_____

_____

_____

_____

_____

_____

_____

TERMS

Objective

- Define the key terms as listed.

Define the following using medical terminology. In the last column, indicate how you would explain the meaning of that term to a patient.

Term		Medical Terminology	Patient's Terminology
(463)	Chvostek's sign		
(462)	Dysphagia		
(457)	Endocrinologist		
(476)	Glycosuria		
(471)	Hirsutism		

Student Name _____

Term		Medical Terminology	Patient's Terminology
(476)	Hyperglycemia		
(469)	Hypocalcemia		
(481)	Hypoglycemia		
(471)	Hypokalemia		
(456)	Idiopathic hyperplasia		
(476)	Ketoacidosis		
(476)	Ketone body		
(481)	Lipodystrophy		
(484)	Neuropathy		
(476)	Polydipsia		
(476)	Polyphagia		
(476)	Polyuria		
(463)	Trousseau's sign		
(459)	Turgor		
(475)	Type 1 diabetes mellitus		
(475)	Type 2 diabetes mellitus		

IMBALANCE

Objective

- Describe the pathophysiology, clinical manifestations, medical management, and nursing interventions of the patient with an imbalance of hormones produced by the anterior and posterior pituitary gland, thyroid, parathyroid, and adrenal glands.

Determine the common etiology/pathophysiology, clinical manifestations, medical management, and nursing interventions for patients with an imbalance of hormones produced by the anterior and posterior pituitary glands, thyroid, parathyroid, or adrenal glands. Then, under each disorder list the specific information that differentiates that imbalance from the others. *(456-474)*

Common

Pathophysiology

Clinical manifestations

Medical management

Nursing interventions

Specific Information

(456)   Anterior and posterior pituitary

(461)   Thyroid

Student Name _____

(461)   Parathyroid

(471)   Adrenal

STRUCTURE OF THE ADRENAL GLANDS

Objective

- List and describe the endocrine glands and their hormones.

Label the parts of the adrenal gland. *(455)*

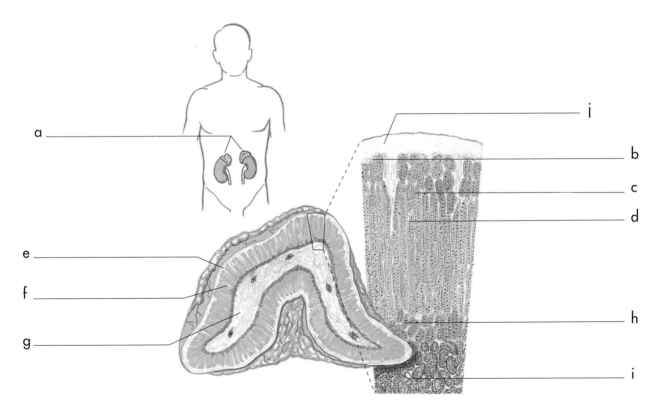

DIABETES INSIPIDUS

Objective

- List four clinical manifestations of diabetes insipidus.

List the clinical manifestations of diabetes insipidus on the lines below. *(458)*

1. _____

2. _____

3. _____

4. _____

MANIFESTATIONS

Objective

- Give the clinical manifestations for patients with acromegaly, giantism, pheochromocytoma, hyper-parathyroidism, and hypoparathyroidism.

Add clinical manifestations of each of the disorders in the space provided.

	Disorders	Clinical Manifestations
(456)	Acromegaly	
(457)	Gigantism	
(473)	Pheochromocytoma	
(469)	Hyperparathyroidism	
(470)	Hympoparathyroidism	

Student Name_____

CUSHING'S SYNDROME AND ADDISON'S DISEASE

Objective

- Differentiate between the clinical manifestations of Cushing's syndrome and those of Addison's disease.

List common clinical manifestations in the top box and the specific manifestations under each disorder. *(471-473)*

Common Manifestations

Cushing's Syndrome   **Addison's Disease**

DIABETES MELLITUS

Objectives

- Describe the pathophysiology and clinical manifestations of diabetes mellitus.
- Describe the difference between type 1 and type 2 diabetes mellitus.

List the pathophysiology and clinical manifestations of type 1 and type 2 diabetes mellitus. *(474-475)*

	Pathophysiology	Clinical Manifestations
Type 1		
Type 2		

HELPFUL INFORMATION

Objective

- Explain the interrelationship of nutrition, exercise, and medication in the control of diabetes mellitus.
- List four nursing interventions that foster self-care in the activities of daily living of the patient with diabetes mellitus.

Develop an index card the will prompt you during your patient teaching for the patient with diabetes mellitus. Include how nutrition, exercise, and medication will help control the disorder. List four nursing interventions that will foster self-care in the activities of daily living for this patient. *(478)*

| |
| |
| |
| |
| |
| |
| |
| |
| |

Student Name_____

INSULIN

Objective

- Describe the proper way to draw up and administer insulin.

List the step to draw up and administer insulin. Be brief and make notes so you will remember the steps.
(481)

Steps
1.
2.
3.
4.
5.
6.
7.
8.
9.
10.
11.
12.
13.
14.
15.
16.
17.
18.
19.
20.

SIGNS OF PROBLEMS

Objective

- Differentiate between the signs and symptoms of diabetic ketoacidosis, hyperglycemic hyperosmolar nonketotic coma, and hypoglycemic reaction.

List the signs and symptoms of diabetic ketoacidosis, hyperglycemic reactions, hyperglycemic hyperosmolar nonketotic coma, and hypoglycemic reactions. *(487)*

Problems	Signs and Symptoms
Diabetic ketoacidosis	
Hyperglycemic reactions	
Hyperglycemic hyperosmolar nonketotic coma	
Hypoglycemic reactions	

CHAPTER

12 Care of the Patient with a Reproductive Disorder

Answer Key: Textbook page references are provided as a guide for answering these questions. A complete answer key was provided for your instructor.

FUNCTIONS

Objective

- List and describe the functions of the organs of the male and female reproductive tracts.

Complete the table below by filling in the functions of the organs of the male and female reproductive tracts.

	Organ	Function
	Male Reproductive Tract	
(495)	Testes	
(495)	Epididymis	
(495)	Ductus deferens (vas deferens)	
(495)	Ejaculatory duct and urethra	
(495)	Accessory glands Seminal vesicles	
(496)	Prostate gland	
(496)	Cowper's gland	
(496)	Urethra and penis	

(continued next page)

Organ	Function
Female Reproductive Tract	
(496) Ovaries	
(496) Fallopian tubes (oviducts)	
(497) Uterus	
(497) Vagina	
(498) External genitalia	
(498) Accessory glands	
(498) Mammary glands	

TERMS

Objective

- Define the key terms as listed.

Define each of the key terms using the space provided. Be sure to use terminology the patient would understand.

(506-507)   1.   Amenorrhea _____

(545)   2.   Candidiasis _____

(524)   3.   Carcinoma in situ _____

(543)   4.   Chancre _____

(545)   5.   *Chlamydia trachomatis* _____

(539)   6.   Cirucumcision _____

Student Name_____

(512)   7.   Climacteric _____

(521)   8.   Colporrhaphy _____

(503)   9.   Colposcopy _____

(540)   10.   Crypotorchidism _____

(503)   11.   Culdoscopy _____

(504)   12.   Curettage _____

(506, 508)   13.   Dysmenorrhea _____

(519)   14.   Endometriosis _____

(539)   15.   Epididymitis _____

(520)   16.   Fistula _____

(521)   17.   Introitus _____

(503)   18.   Laparoscopy _____

(531)   19.   Mammography _____

(506, 508)   20.   Menorrhagia _____

(508)   21.   Metrorrhagia _____

(527)   22.   Panhysterosalpingo-oophorectomy _____

(503)   23.   Papanicolaou test (smear) _____

(539)   24.   Phimosis _____

(521)   25.   Procidentia _____

(531)   26.   Sentinel lymph node mapping _____

(544)   27.   Trichomoniasis _____

SEXUALITY

Objective

- Discuss the impact of illness on the patient's sexuality.

Develop an index card listing how illness may affect a patient's sexuality. *(500-502)*

<table>
<tr><td></td></tr>
<tr><td></td></tr>
<tr><td></td></tr>
<tr><td></td></tr>
<tr><td></td></tr>
<tr><td></td></tr>
<tr><td></td></tr>
<tr><td></td></tr>
<tr><td></td></tr>
<tr><td></td></tr>
<tr><td></td></tr>
</table>

MENSTRUAL DISTURBANCES

Objective

- List nursing interventions for patients with menstrual disturbances.

Next to each disturbance of menstruation, list appropriate nursing interventions.

	Disturbances	Nursing Interventions
(506, 507)	Amenorrhea	
(506, 508)	Dysmenorrhea	
(506, 508)	Abnormal uterine bleeding Menorrhagia	
(508)	Metrorrhagia	

Student Name_____

DIAGNOSTIC STUDIES

Objective

- Discuss nursing interventions for the patient undergoing diagnostic studies related to the reproductive system.

Your patient is undergoing a diagnostic study for a problem related to her reproductive system. List what patient teaching you will initiate, the assessment you will do, and actions you will carry out for your patient. *(506)*

Activity	Responses
Patient teaching	1.
	2.
	3.
	4.
	5.
	6.
	7.
	8.
	9.
	10.
Assessment	1.
	2.
	3.
Actions	1.
	2.
	3.

SECTIONAL VIEW OF THE UTERUS

Objective

- List and describe the functions of the organs of the male and female reproductive tracts.

Label the parts of the female reproductive organs. *(497)*

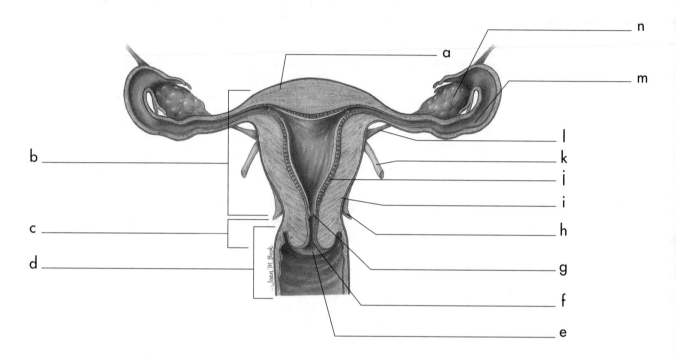

PAP SMEAR

Objective

- Discuss the importance of the Papanicolaou smear test in early detection of cervical cancer.

Your patient, a teenager, is in for her first Pap smear. Explain to her what the American Cancer Society recommends for all women about early detection of cervical cancer and why. *(503)*

Student Name _____

PID

Objective

- Discuss four important points to be addressed in discharge planning for the patient with pelvic inflammatory disease (PID).

Develop a short checklist of four important points to include in discharge planning for the patient with PID. *(518)*

1 . _____

2 . _____

3 . _____

4 . _____

ENDOMETRIOSIS

Objective

- List four nursing diagnoses pertinent to the patient with endometriosis.

In the space provided, identify four nursing diagnoses pertinent to your patient who has endometriosis. *(520)*

1. _____

2. _____

3. _____

4. _____

FISTULA

Objective

- Identify the clinical manifestations of a vaginal fistula.

List the clinical manifestations for a patient with a vagina fistula. *(520)*

SURGERY

Objective

- Describe the preoperative and postoperative nursing interventions for the patient requiring major surgery of the female reproductive system.

Develop an index card to use to prompt you during your care of the patient who requires major surgery of the female reproductive system. *(527-528)*

<table>
<tr><td></td></tr>
<tr><td></td></tr>
<tr><td></td></tr>
<tr><td></td></tr>
<tr><td></td></tr>
<tr><td></td></tr>
<tr><td></td></tr>
<tr><td></td></tr>
<tr><td></td></tr>
<tr><td></td></tr>
</table>

Student Name _____

CYSTOCELE AND RECTOCELE

Objective

- Describe the common problems of cystocele, rectocele, and the related medical management and nursing interventions.

Fill in the chain of events below for the patient with a cystocele or rectocele. *(522)*

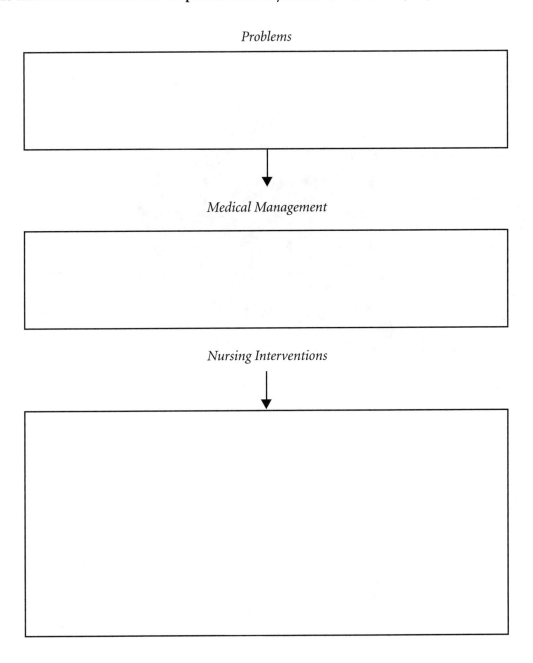

Problems

Medical Management

Nursing Interventions

LONGITUDINAL SECTION OF THE MALE PENIS

Objective

- List and describe the functions of the organs of the male and female reproductive tracts.

Label the parts of the male reproductive organs. *(495)*

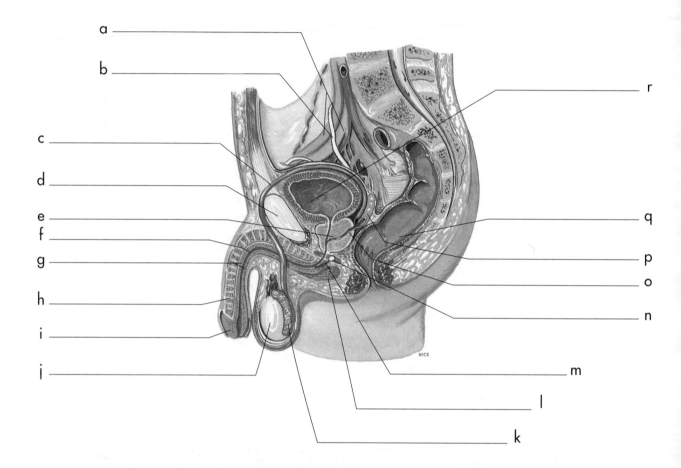

Student Name _____

PROSTATITIS

Objective

- Describe nursing interventions for the patient with prostatitis.

List the nursing interventions for your patient with prostatitis. *(538)*

1. _____

2. _____

3. _____

    a. _____

    b. _____

    c. _____

    d. _____

4. _____

5. _____

6. _____

TESTICULAR SELF-EXAMINATION

Objective

- Discuss the importance of monthly testicular self-examination beginning at 15 years of age.

You have a 16-year-old male in the office for his annual exam. Explain to him the need for him to do a monthly testicular self-examination. *(540)*

CHAPTER 13

Care of the Patient with a Sensory Disorder

Answer Key: Textbook page references are provided as a guide for answering these questions. A complete answer key was provided for your instructor.

SENSORY ORGANS

Objectives

- List the major sense organs and discuss their anatomical position.
- List the parts of the eye and define the function of each part.
- List the three divisions of the ear, and discuss the function of each.

Next to each sensory organ, list its anatomical position and function.

	Sensory Organ	Anatomical Position	Function
	Eye		
(556)	Lacrimal apparatus		
(556)	Conjunctiva		
(556)	Extrinsic eye muscles		
(557)	Sclera		
(557)	Cornea		
(557)	Choroid		
(557)	Pupil		
(557)	Retina		

(continued next page)

	Sensory Organ	Anatomical Position	Function
(557)	Rods and cones		
(557)	Crystalline lens		
(557)	Aqueous humor		
(557)	Vitreous humor		

Ear – External

(558)	Tympanic membrane		
(558)	Ceruminous glands		

Ear – Middle

(558)	Eustachian tube		
(558)	Ossicles		

Ear – Inner

(559)	Labyrinth 1.　Semicircular canal		
	2.　Vestibule		
	3.　Cochlea		
(559)	Cochlea nerve		
(559)	Vestibule nerve		

Student Name _____

TERMS

Objective

- Define the key terms as listed.

Match the correct definition to the term by placing the letter of the definition next to the term.

		Terms	Matching Letter		Definitions
(561, 565)	1.	Astigmatism	_____	A.	An abnormal condition characterized by a marked protrusion of the eyeballs
(585)	2.	Audiometry	_____	B.	Diagnostic test to screen for visual abnormalities
(570)	3.	Cataract	_____	C.	Defect in the curvature of the eyeball surface
(567)	4.	Conjunctivitis	_____	D.	Inability of the eyes to focus in the same direction; cross-eyed
(575)	5.	Cryosurgery	_____	E.	Condition of nearsightedness
(572)	6.	Diabetic retinopathy	_____	F.	Condition of farsightedness
(582)	7.	Enucleation	_____	G.	A technique in which the surgeon makes partial-thickness, radial incisions in the patient's cornea
(562)	8.	Exophthalmos	_____	H.	An inflammation of the conjunctiva caused by bacterial or viral infection
(576)	9.	Glaucoma	_____	I.	An inflammation of the cornea resulting from injury
(561, 565)	10.	Hyperopia	_____	J.	Corneal transplant
(568)	11.	Keratitis	_____	K.	Causing papillary dilation
(582)	12.	Keratoplasty	_____	L.	A disorder of retinal blood vessels characterized by capillary microaneurysms, hemorrhage, exudates, and formation of new vessels
(591)	13.	Labryrinthitis	_____	M.	Separation of the retina from the choroids in the posterior area of the eye
(590)	14.	Mastoiditis	_____	N.	An abnormal condition of elevated pressure within the eye because of obstruction of the outflow of aqueous humor
(577)	15.	Miotic	_____	O.	Agents that cause the pupil to contract
(562)	16.	Mydriatic	_____	P.	Surgical removal of the eyeball

(continued next page)

		Terms	Matching Letter		Definitions
(561, 565)	17.	Myopia	_____	Q.	The excision of the corneal tissue followed by surgical implantation of a cornea from another human donor
(596)	18.	Myringotomy	_____	R.	Test of hearing acuity
(565)	19.	Radial keratotomy	_____	S.	An infection of one of the mastoid bones
(574)	20.	Retinal detachment	_____	T.	An inflammation of the labyrinthine canals of the inner ear
(569)	21.	Sjogren's syndrome	_____	U.	Sensation that the outer world is revolving about oneself or that one is moving in space
(561)	22.	Snellen test	_____	V.	The removal of the stapes of the middle ear and insertion of graft and prosthesis
(594)	23.	Stapedectomy	_____	W.	Operative procedure on the eardrum or ossicles of the middle ear designed to improve hearing in patients with conductive hearing loss
(565)	24.	Strabismus	_____	X.	Surgical incision of the eardrum
(588)	25.	Tinnitus	_____	Y.	Used to freeze the borders of a retinal hole with a frozen-tipped probe
(595)	26.	Tympanoplasty	_____	Z.	Subjective noise sensation heard in one or both ears; ringing or tinkling sounds in the ear.
(591)	27.	Vertigo	_____	AA.	Dry eye in patients with keratoconjunctivitis sicca

AGING

Objectives

- Describe two changes in the sensory system that occur as a result of the normal aging process.
- Describe age-related changes in the visual and auditory systems and differences in assessment findings.

Develop a patient teaching tool that highlights the changes in the sensory system because of the normal aging process. *(560)*

Student Name

DIAGNOSTIC STUDIES

Objective

- Describe the purpose, significance of results, and nursing responsibilities related to diagnostic studies of the visual and auditory systems.

Complete the following table of diagnostic studies by including the purpose, significance of the abnormal results, and nursing interventions for each.

	Diagnostic Study	Purpose	Abnormal Result Significance	Nursing Interventions
(561)	Snellen test			
(561)	Color vision			
(561)	Refraction			
(562)	Ophthalmoscopy			
(562)	Tonometry			
(562)	Amsler grid test			
(562)	Schirmer's tear test			
(584)	Otoscopy			
(584)	Tuning fork			
(584)	Audiometry			
(584)	Vestibular testing			

LACRIMAL APPARATUS

Objective

- List the major sense organs and discuss their anatomical position.

Identify each part of the lacrimal apparatus. *(556)*

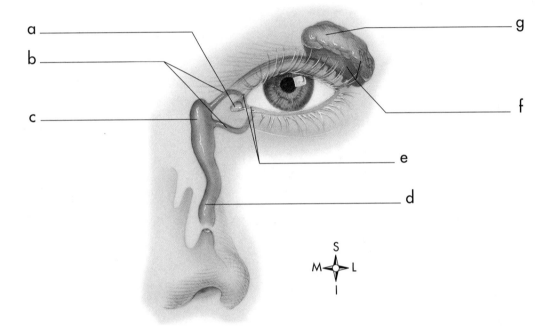

Student Name_____

HORIZONTAL SECTION OF THE EYEBALL

Objective

- List the parts of the eye and define the function of each part.

Label the parts of the eyeball. *(556)*

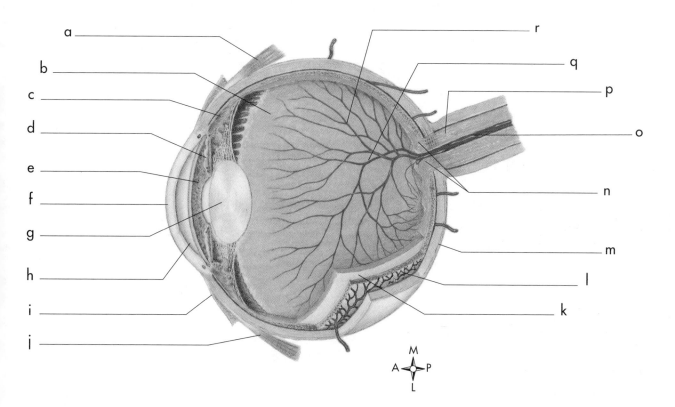

TREATMENT OF THE EYE AND EAR

Objectives

- Identify the nursing interventions associated with medical-surgical treatments of the eye and ear.
- Describe appropriate nursing interventions for the patient having eye and ear surgery.

Your patient had a car accident and is returning to your unit from vitrectomy surgery of the right eye and a myringotomy of the right ear. List the appropriate nursing interventions for this patient. *(583, 597)*

HEARING LOSS

Objective

- Differentiate between conductive and sensorineural hearing loss.

List the common characteristics of conductive and sensorineural hearing loss in the center column. In other columns below, list specific information about conductive and sensorineural hearing loss. *(585)*

Conductive Hearing Loss	Common Characteristics	Sensorineural Hearing Loss

PATIENT TEACHING

Objective

- Give patient instructions regarding care of the eye and ear in accordance with written protocol.

Develop an index card to use to prompt you during patient teaching for care of the eye and ear in accordance with written protocol. *(573, 595)*

CHAPTER 14
Care of the Patient with a Neurological Disorder

Answer Key: Textbook page references are provided as a guide for answering these questions. A complete answer key was provided for your instructor.

NEURON

Objective

- List the parts of the neuron, and describe the function of each part.

Identify each part of the neuron. Next to each label describe the function of that part. *(602)*

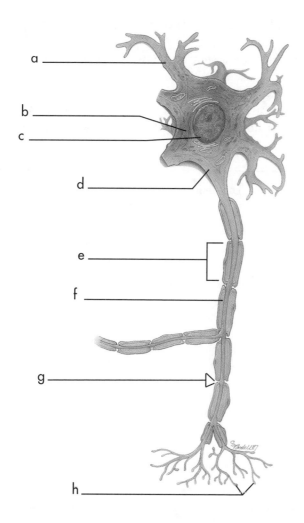

a _____

b _____

c _____

d _____

e _____

f _____

g _____

h _____

Describe the function of each part.

a. _____

b. _____

c. _____

d. _____

e. _____

f. _____

g. _____

h. _____

NERVOUS SYSTEM

Objectives

- Explain the anatomical location and functions of the cerebrum, brainstem, cerebellum, spinal cord, peripheral nerves, and cerebrospinal fluid.
- Discuss the parts of the peripheral nervous system and how the system works with the central nervous system (CNS).

Complete the table below with the anatomical location and function of the cerebrum, brainstem, cerebellum, spinal cord, peripheral nerves (include how they work with the central nervous system), and cerebrospinal fluid.

	Part	Location	Function
(603)	Cerebrum		
(604)	Brainstem		
(603)	Cerebellum		
(605)	Spinal cord		
(605)	Peripheral nerves		

Student Name_____

CRANIAL NERVES

Objective

- Name the 12 cranial nerves, and list the areas they serve.

Develop a method of remembering the 12 cranial nerves and the areas they serve and describe it in the space provided. *(606, 608)*

TERMS

Objective

- Define the key terms as listed.

Define the following terms using medical terminology. In the last column, indicate how you would explain the meaning of that term to a patient.

	Term	Medical Terminology	Patient's Terminology
(622)	Agnosia		
(638)	Aneurysm		
(608)	Aphasia		
(633)	Apraxia		
(626)	Ataxia		
(624)	Aura		
(628)	Bradykinesia		

(continued next page)

	Term	Medical Terminology	Patient's Terminology
(616)	Diplopia		
(608)	Dysarthria		
(620)	Dysphagia		
(608)	Flaccid		
(607)	Glasgow coma scale		
(647)	Global cognitive dysfunction		
(609)	Hemianopia		
(620)	Hemiplegia		
(650)	Hyperreflexia		
(626)	Nystagmus		
(608)	Paresis		
(624)	Postictal period		
(609)	Proprioception		
(608)	Spastic		
(609)	Unilateral neglect		

AGING

Objective

- List the physiological changes that occur in the nervous system with aging.

Develop a fact sheet about changes to the nervous system that occur with aging. *(606)*

Brain weight _____

Structural changes _____

Neuron changes _____

Body function changes _____

Student Name_____

GLASGOW COMA SCALE

Objective

- Discuss Glasgow coma scale.

Complete the table below to use as a guide when you are assessing a patient's level of consciousness. *(607, 608)*

Response	Score
Eyes open	
Verbal	
Motor	
Total	

NEUROLOGICAL RESPONSE TO TRAUMA

Objective

- Identify the significant subjective and objective data related to the nervous system that should be obtained from a patient during assessment.

Indicate the type of neurological response each patient is exhibiting. *(617)*

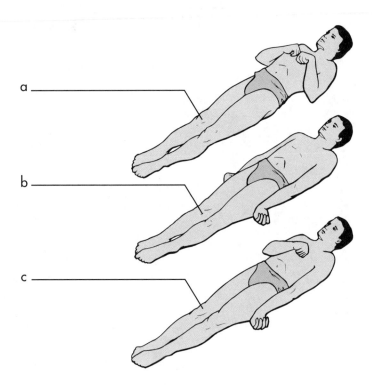

a _____

b _____

c _____

Student Name _____

ASSESSMENT

Objectives

- Identify the significant subjective and objective data related to the nervous system that should be obtained from a patient during assessment.
- Differentiate between normal and common abnormal findings of a physical assessment of the nervous system.

Your patient has just arrived on the unit after falling from the roof of his house and sustaining a head injury. During your data collection of his nervous system what normal and abnormal subjective and objective data could be obtained from your patient? List possible abnormal and normal findings below. *(607-608)*

Assessment	Normal Findings	Abnormal Findings
History		
Mental status		
Level of consciousness		
Language and speech		
Cranial nerves		
Motor function		
Sensory and perceptual status		

PREVENTION

Objective

- Explain the importance of prevention in problems of the nervous system, and give at least one example of prevention.

Your patient has asked you what she could do to reduce her risk factors that may contribute to a neurological problem. Explain below what you would tell her. Be sure to list at least one example. *(606-607)*

INTRACRANIAL PRESSURE (ICP)

Objective

- List five signs and symptoms of increased intracranial pressure and why they occur, as well as nursing interventions that decrease intracranial pressure.

Identify five signs and symptoms of ICP and why they occur. Then list nursing interventions that would assist in decreasing ICP. *(616-618)*

Signs and Symptoms	Nursing Interventions
1.	
2.	
3.	
4.	
5.	

Student Name _____

STROKE

Objectives

- Explain the mechanism of injury to the brain that occurs with a stroke and traumatic brain injury.
- Describe the medical management of the acute stroke patient.
- Discuss nursing interventions to assist in the rehabilitation of the patient with a stroke.
- Describe the acute nursing interventions of the stroke patient.

Complete the chain of events for a patient who has suffered a stroke or a traumatic brain injury. *(637-642)*

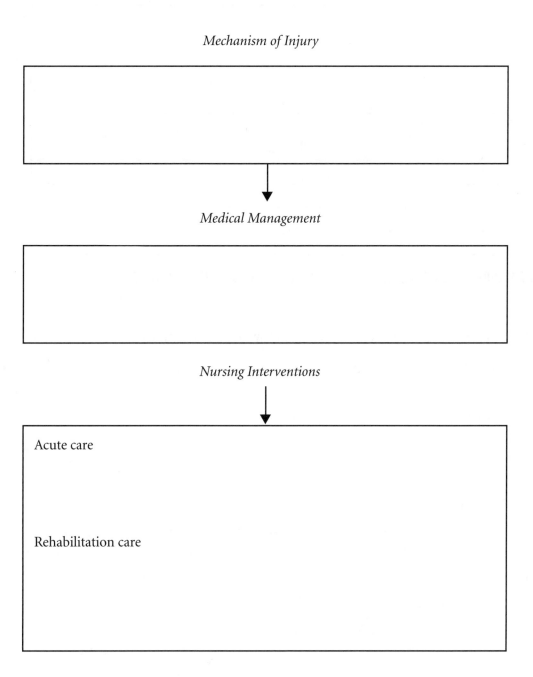

Mechanism of Injury

Medical Management

Nursing Interventions

Acute care

Rehabilitation care

MS, PARKINSON'S, MYASTHENIA GRAVIS

Objective

- Discuss patient teaching and home care planning for the patient with multiple sclerosis (MS), Parkinson's disease, and myasthenia gravis.

Prepare an index card that has patient teaching and home care planning for patients with MS, Parkinson's disease, and myasthenia gravis. *(626-632, 634-636)*

GUILLAIN-BARRÉ SYNDROME, TRIGEMINAL NEURALGIA, AND BELL'S PALSY.

Objective

- Discuss the pathophysiology of Guillain-Barré syndrome, trigeminal neuralgia, and Bell's palsy.

List the pathophysiology of Guillain-Barré syndrome, trigeminal neuralgia, and Bell's palsy. *(642-645)*

Guillain-Barré syndrome

Trigeminal neuralgia

Bell's palsy

CHAPTER 15

Care of the Patient with an Immune Disorder

Answer Key: Textbook page references are provided as a guide for answering these questions. A complete answer key was provided for your instructor.

TERMS

Objective

- Define the key terms as listed.

Develop sentences for a patient teaching presentation using the following key terms. You may combine more than one term in a sentence and have more than one topic in your presentation. Be sure that your patient will understand the meaning of each word.

(658)	Adaptive immunity	*(657)*	Immunocompetence
(659)	Allergen	*(666)*	Immunodeficiency
(659)	Antigen	*(659)*	Immunogen
(661)	Attenuated	*(657)*	Immunology
(667)	Autoimmune	*(665)*	Immunosuppressive
(665)	Autologous	*(661)*	Immunotherapy
(660)	Cellular immunity	*(658)*	Innate immunity
(659)	Humoral immunity	*(659)*	Lymphokine
(662)	Hypersensitivity	*(667)*	Plasmapheresis
(657)	Immunity	*(659)*	Proliferation
(659)	Immunization		

_____

_____

_____

_____

_____

_____

_____

_____

_____

_____

_____

_____

_____

_____

_____

_____

_____

ORGANIZATION OF THE IMMUNE SYSTEM

Objective

- Review the mechanisms of immune response.

Identify the location of the immune organs. *(658)*

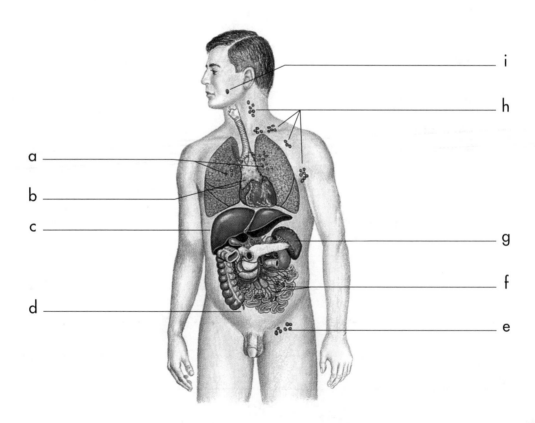

Student Name _____

IMMUNITY

Objective

- Differentiate between natural and acquired immunity.

List the purpose and pathophysiology of natural and acquired immunity. *(658-659)*

	Purpose	Pathophysiology
Natural immunity		
Acquired immunity		

IMMUNITY DIFFERENCES

Objective

- Explain the concepts of immunocompetency, immunodeficiency, and autoimmunity.

Your patient has asked you to explain the differences among immunocompetency, immunodeficiency, and autoimmunity. She said that she had written these three words down, but doesn't have any idea what they mean. Explain the differences to her in terms she can understand. *(666-667)*

ANAPHYLAXIS

Objectives

- Identify the clinical manifestations of anaphylaxis.
- Outline the immediate aggressive treatment of systemic anaphylactic reaction.

List the body system and the sign that would indicate that your patient may be having an anaphylactic response. In the last row, outline the treatment of a systemic anaphylactic reaction. *(664-665)*

System	Sign
1.	
2.	
3.	
4.	
Treatment	

TRANSFUSION REACTION

Objective

- Discuss selection of blood donors, typing and cross-matching, storage, and administration in the prevention of transfusion reaction.

Complete the index card below to outline information about preventing transfusion reactions to assist you in caring for a patient receiving a blood transfusion. *(665-666)*

Selection of blood donors
Typing and cross-matching
Storage of blood
Administration of blood

Student Name_____

AUTOIMMUNE DISORDERS

Objectives

- Discuss the causation of autoimmune disorders; explain plasmapheresis in the treatment of autoimmune diseases.

Your patient has an autoimmune disorder. Explain to him what could be the possible causes of autoimmune disorders and how plasmapheresis treatment will be helpful. *(667)*

IMMUNODEFICIENCY DISEASE

Objective

- Explain an immunodeficiency disease.

Complete the chart below that depicts an immunodeficency disease. *(666)*

First evidence:

Result of immunodeficient state:

Two types:

1. _____

2. _____

Factors that alter immune response:

1. _____

2 _____

3. _____

4. _____

CHAPTER 16 Care of the Patient with HIV/AIDS

Answer Key: Textbook page references are provided as a guide for answering these questions. A complete answer key was provided for your instructor.

TERMS

Objective

- Define the key terms as listed.

Define each of the key terms in the space provided. Use terminology that your patient would understand.

	Term	Definition
(680)	Acquired immunodeficiency syndrome (AIDS)	
(694)	Adherence	
(679)	CD_4 + lymphocyte	
(670)	Centers for Disease Control	
(675)	Enzyme-linked immuno-sorbent assay (ELISA)	
(680)	HIV disease	
(680)	HIV infection	
(671)	Human immunodeficiency virus	

(continued next page)

Term	Definition
(670) Kaposi's sarcoma	
(671) Opportunistic	
(679) Phagocytic	
(670) *Pneumocystis carinii* pneumonia (PCP)	
(677) Retrovirus	
(675) Seroconversion	
(682) Seronegative	
(674) Vertical transmission	
(674) Viral load	
(671) Virulent	
(675) Western blot	

CAUSE OF HIV

Objectives

- Describe the agent that causes HIV disease.
- Describe definition of AIDS given in January 1993 by the Centers for Disease Control and Prevention.
- Explain the differences between HIV infection, HIV disease, and AIDS.
- Define the nurse's role in the prevention of HIV infection.

Student Name_____

You are instructing a young male patient about HIV disease and the differences among HIV infection, HIV disease, and AIDS. Develop information that you can share with him about this disease, including the definition of AIDS that the Centers of Disease Control and Prevention gave in January 1993. After you have developed this information, describe your role in prevention of HIV infection. *(670-674)*

VIRAL LOAD IN THE BLOOD

Objective

- Describe the progression of HIV infection.

Label the significance of viral load in the blood and months of the disease. *(674)*

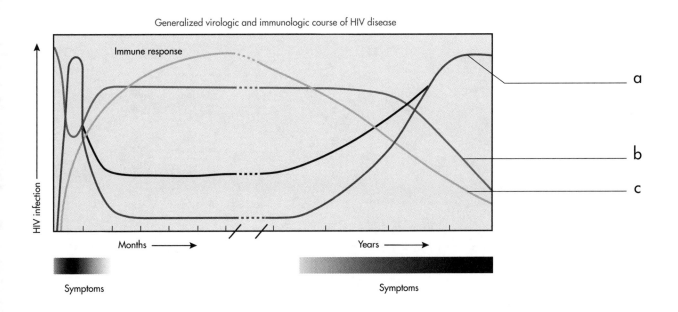

210

000

000

000

DIAGNOSTIC TESTS

Objective

- Discuss the laboratory and diagnostic tests related to HIV disease.

Complete the following table about diagnostic tests used to determine your patient's status with HIV disease.

	Diagnostic Test	Implications and Process
(682)	HIV antibody testing	
	1.	
	2.	
	3.	
	4.	
	5.	
(682)	CD_4 + cell monitoring	
(683)	Viral load monitoring	
(684)	CBC	
(684)	Liver function	
(684)	Syphilis	

Student Name_____

COMMON CLINICAL CONDITIONS

Objective

- List signs and symptoms that may be indicative of HIV disease.

Identify the significance of CD_4 + lymphocyte and months of the disease. *(684)*

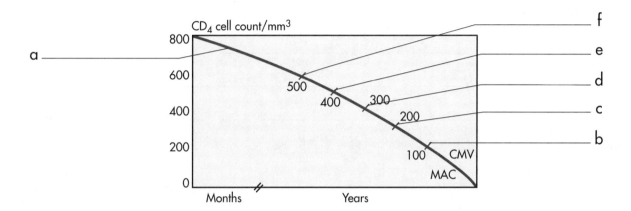

RISK FOR HIV

Objectives

- Describe patients who are at risk for HIV infection.
- Discuss the use of effective prevention messages in counseling patients.

Identify patients who are at risk for HIV infections in the column to the left. In the column on the right, describe use of effective prevention messages. *(675-677)*

Patients at Risk	Effective Prevention Messages

ISSUES WITH TESTING

Objective

- Discuss the issues related to HIV antibody testing.

Prepare a short checklist of topics that you would include when counseling a patient about HIV antibody testing. Include general guidelines and pretest and post-test counseling. *(683)*

General Guidelines

1. _____

2. _____

3. _____

Pretest Counseling

1. _____

2. _____

3. _____

4. _____

5. _____

6. _____

7. _____

8. _____

9. _____

10. _____

Post-test Counseling

1. _____

2. _____

Student Name_____

NURSE'S ROLE

Objective

- Discuss the nurse's role in assisting the HIV-infected patient with coping, grieving, reducing anxiety, and minimizing social isolation.

Make an index card of helpful information about coping, grieving, reducing anxiety, and minimizing social isolation to assist you during your care of an HIV-infected patient. *(695)*

| |
| |

MULTIDISCIPLINARY CARE

Objective

- Describe the multidisciplinary approach in caring for a patient with HIV disease.

Your patient wants to know why she has so many doctors and nurses in her room all the time. Explain to her the multidisciplinary approach that is being utilized in her care. *(685)*

ADHERENCE TO TREATMENT

Objective

- Discuss the importance of adherence to HIV treatment.

Your patient says that she was only taking two pills before she was told she has HIV. She doesn't understand why she will have to take all of those pills once she goes home. Prepare a short information sheet with facts related to nonadherent behavior that will help you in explaining to your patient why it is important to follow recommended treatment. *(695)*

Factor	Examples
Psychosocial factors	
Medications and treatments	
Cultural issues	
Substance use	

OPPORTUNISTIC INFECTIONS

Objective

- List opportunistic infections associated with advanced HIV disease (AIDS).

List the opportunistic infections that your patient may develop because of advanced HIV disease. List the infections under each system and then list common symptoms that would alert you to the possibility that your patient has an opportunistic infection.

	System	Opportunistic Infections
(685)	Respiratory	
(686)	Integumentary	

_____

(686)   Eye

(686)   Gastrointestinal

(687)   Neurological

_____

CARE PLAN

Objective

- Implement a care plan for the patient with AIDS.

You have been assigned to a patient who has AIDS. Since nursing care is complex and constant, make a list of care that you would give and goals that you would promote. *(692-694)*

CHAPTER

17 Care of the Patient with Cancer

Answer Key: Textbook page references are provided as a guide for answering these questions. A complete answer key was provided for your instructor.

TERMS

Objective

- Define the key terms as listed.

Match the correct definition to the term by placing the letter of the definition next to the term.

		Terms	Matching Letter		Definitions
(729)	1.	Alopecia	_____	A.	The sum of knowledge regarding tumors; a branch of medicine that deals with the study of tumors
(733)	2.	Autologous	_____	B.	Substances known to increase the risk for the development of cancer
(717)	3.	Benign	_____	C.	A pelvic examination for women to detect cancer
(720)	4.	Biopsy	_____	D.	Radiographic study of the breast
(713)	5.	Carcinogen	_____	E.	Not recurrent or progressive; nonmalignant
(713)	6.	Carcinogenesis	_____	F.	Growing worse and resisting treatment
(718)	7.	Carcinoma	_____	G.	The process by which tumor cells are spread to distant parts of the body
(719)	8.	Differentiated	_____	H.	The immune system's recognition and destruction of newly developed abnormal cells
(718)	9.	Immuno-surveillance	_____	I.	Term used for malignant tumors composed of epithelial cells, which have a tendency to metastasize
(726)	10.	Leukopenia	_____	J.	Loss of hair

(continued next page)

	Terms	Matching Letter		Definitions
(717)	11. Malignant	_____	K.	The term for uncontrolled or abnormal growth of cells
(718)	12. Metastasis	_____	L.	A reduction in the number of circulating platelets due to the suppression of the bone marrow
(717)	13. Neoplasm	_____	M.	A mouth inflammation due to destruction of normal cells of the oval cavity
(712)	14. Oncology	_____	N.	Refers to malignant tumors of connective tissues such as muscle or bone
(722)	15. Palliative	_____	O.	Oncologic emergency that occurs with rapid lysis of malignant cells
(719)	16. Papanicolaou smear	_____	P.	Profound state of ill health, malnutrition, and wasting
(718)	17. Sarcoma	_____	Q.	The process by which normal cells are transformed into cancer cells
(729)	18. Stomatitis	_____	R.	Most like the parent tissue
(729)	19. Thrombo-cytopenia	_____	S.	Reduction in the number of circulating white blood cells due to depression of the bone marrow
(732)	20. Tumor lysis syndrome	_____	T.	Indicating something that has its origin within an individual, especially a factor present in tissues or fluids
		_____	U.	Removal of a small piece of living tissue from an organ or other part of the body for microscopic examination
		_____	V.	Therapy designed to relieve or reduce intensity of uncomfortable symptoms; does not produce a cure

Student Name _____

PREVENTION AND DETECTION

Objectives

- Discuss development, prevention, and detection of cancer.
- Explain common reasons for delay in seeking medical care when a diagnosis of cancer is suspected.

Develop a chart below to explain how cancer develops, how it can be prevented, detected, and common reasons for delaying seeking medical care. Prepare this so that a young adult would be interested in hearing your remarks. *(714-719)*

MALIGNANT CELLS

Objectives

- Define the terminology used to describe cellular changes, characteristics of malignant cells, and types of malignancies.
- Describe the pathophysiology of cancer, including the characteristics of malignant cells and the nature of metastasis.
- Describe the process of metastasis.

Describe cellular changes and pathophysiology and characteristics of malignant cells and list the types of malignancies in the box below. In the bottom box, explain the process of metastasis. *(716-720)*

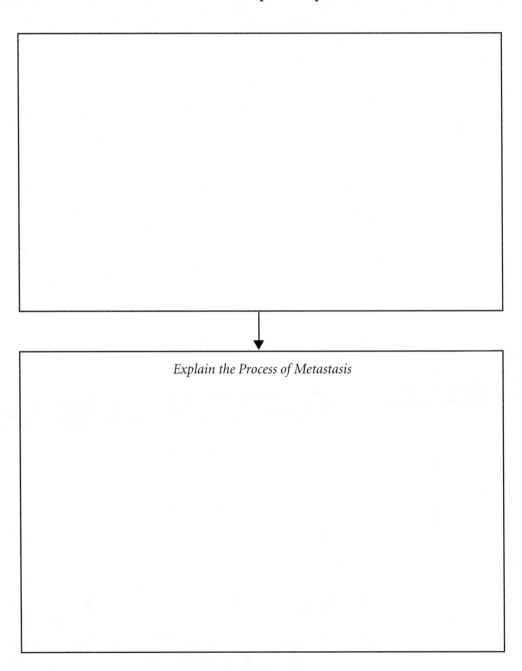

Explain the Process of Metastasis

Student Name_____

CHEMOTHERAPEUTIC AGENTS

Objective

- Describe the major categories of chemotherapeutic agents.

Prepare a hint sheet of six major categories of chemotherapeutic agents. Include mode of action and common side effects that you would need to know if you are taking care of a patient receiving this type of treatment. *(727)*

Categories	Mode of Action and Common Side Effects
1.	
2.	
3.	
4.	
5.	
6.	

DIAGNOSTIC TESTS

Objective

- List common diagnostic tests used to identify the presence of cancer.

Complete the table below listing diagnostic tests and the purpose of each.

	Diagnostic Test	Purpose
(720)	Biopsy	
(720-721)	Endoscopy	
(721)	Bone scanning	
(721)	Computed tomography	
(721)	Ultrasound tests	
(721)	Magnetic resonance imaging	
(721)	Alkaline phosphatase	
(721)	Serum calcitonin	
(721)	Carcinoembryonic antigen	
(721)	PSA and CA-125	
(722)	Stool examination	

Student Name _____

TYPES OF BIOPSY

Objective

- List common diagnostic tests used to identify the presence of cancer.

Label each type of biopsy. *(720)*

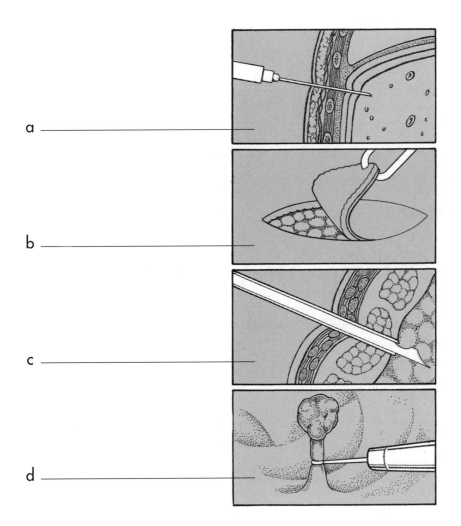

a _____

b _____

c _____

d _____

PAIN

Objective

- Discuss six general guidelines for the use of pain relief measures for the patient with advanced cancer.

List the six guidelines for use in pain relief. *(734)*

1. _____

2. _____

3. _____

4. _____

5. _____

6. _____

NURSING INTERVENTIONS

Objective

- Describe nursing interventions for the individual undergoing surgery, radiation therapy, chemotherapy, bone marrow, or peripheral stem cell transplantation.

Make an index card that you can use listing nursing interventions for the patient undergoing surgery, radiation therapy, chemotherapy, or bone marrow or peripheral stem cell transplant. *(733-734)*

Student Name_____

TUMOR LYSIS SYNDROME

Objective

- Explain the pathophysiology of and medical management and nursing intervention for tumor lysis syndrome.

Complete the flow chart below, explaining the pathophysiology, medical management, and nursing interventions for tumor lysis syndrome. *(732)*

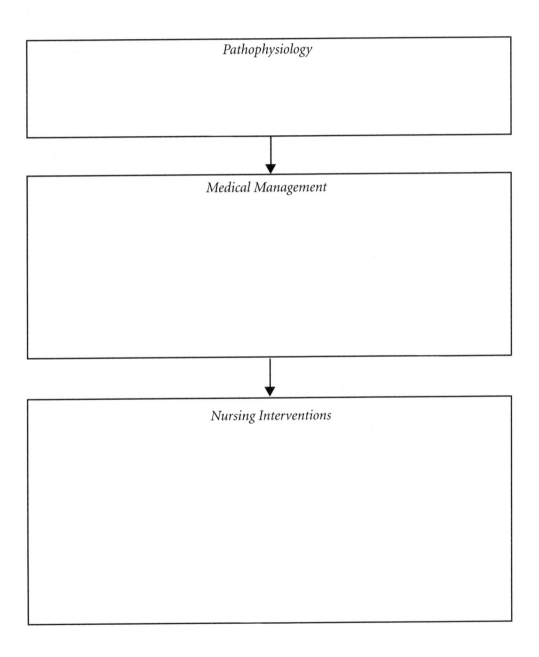

Pathophysiology

Medical Management

Nursing Interventions

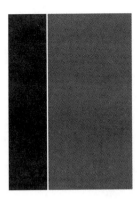

Skills Performance Checklists

These checklists were developed to assist in evaluating the competence of students in performing the nursing interventions presented in the text *Adult Health Nursing*. The checklists are perforated for easy removal and reference. Students can be evaluated with a "Satisfactory" or "Unsatisfactory" performance rating by putting a check in the appropriate column for each step. Specific instruction or feedback can be provided in the "Comments" column. All the checklists have been streamlined to include **only** the critical steps needed to satisfactorily master the skill. They are **not** intended to replace the text, which describes and illustrates each nursing skill in detail.

Student Name _____ Date _____ Instructor's Name _____

PERFORMANCE CHECKLIST 2-1

Performing a Surgical Skin Preparation

		S	U	Comments
1.	Wash hands	❏	❏	_____
2.	Refer to medical record, care plan, or Kardex for special interventions	❏	❏	_____
3.	Refer to procedure manual to verify anatomical area to be shaved according to surgery to be performed	❏	❏	_____
4.	Obtain equipment	❏	❏	_____
5.	Close door, pull curtains	❏	❏	_____
6.	Explain procedure to patient	❏	❏	_____
7.	Position bed and patient	❏	❏	_____
8.	Place towel or waterproof pad under area to be shaved	❏	❏	_____
9.	Fill basin with warm water	❏	❏	_____
10.	Use bath blanket to drape patient appropriately to limit exposure	❏	❏	_____
11.	Adjust lighting	❏	❏	_____
12.	Don gloves	❏	❏	_____
13.	Lather skin well with antiseptic soap or lather and warm water using gauze squares	❏	❏	_____
14.	Hold razor at a 30- to 45-degree angle to skin	❏	❏	_____
	a. Shave small area at a time while holding skin taut	❏	❏	_____
	b. Use short, smooth strokes	❏	❏	_____
	c. Shave hair in direction it grows	❏	❏	_____

		S	U	Comments
15.	Rinse razor frequently	❏	❏	_____
	a. Change blade as needed; replace razor, if disposable razor is used	❏	❏	_____
	b. Change water as needed	❏	❏	_____
	c. Cleanse navel area with sterile, cotton-tipped applicators	❏	❏	_____
16.	When entire area is shaved, use washcloth and clean, warm water to cleanse area; dry skin	❏	❏	_____
17.	Reassess skin for cuts, abrasions, or hair	❏	❏	_____
18.	Return patient to comfortable status	❏	❏	_____
19.	Clean and dispose of equipment	❏	❏	_____
20.	Remove gloves and dispose of in proper receptacle	❏	❏	_____
21.	Wash hands	❏	❏	_____
22.	Often a patient is asked to shower with an antiseptic soap, such as Hibiclens, after the surgical shave or prep to remove any hair and for further cleansing	❏	❏	_____
23.	Document and do patient teaching	❏	❏	_____

Student Name _____ Date _____ Instructor's Name _____

PERFORMANCE CHECKLIST 2-2

INCENTIVE SPIROMETRY

		S	U	Comments
1.	Check the physician's orders, care plan, or Kardex	❏	❏	_____
2.	Assess patient's respiratory status and lung sounds. Indicators for spirometry are: a. asymmetrical chest wall movement b. increased respiratory rate c. increased production of sputum d. diminished lung expansion e. decreased oxygen saturation f. prevention of postoperative pneumonia g. prevention of atelectasis	❏	❏	_____
3.	Explain procedure, and instruct patient in the correct use of the spirometer (frequently this is initially done by the respiratory therapist)	❏	❏	_____
4.	Obtain supplies and equipment	❏	❏	_____
5.	Wash hands and don gloves (if soiling is likely)	❏	❏	_____
6.	Place prescribed incentive spirometer at the bedside within easy reach of patient	❏	❏	_____
7.	Place patient in semi-Fowler's or full Fowler's position	❏	❏	_____
8.	Place tissues, emesis basin, and bedside trash bag within easy reach	❏	❏	_____
9.	Respiratory therapist will determine patient's inspiratory rate based on age, height, and sex	❏	❏	_____
10.	Instruct patient to completely cover mouthpiece with lips	❏	❏	_____
11.	Instruct patient to (a) inhale slowly until maximum inspiration is reached, (b) hold breath 2 or 3 seconds, and (c) slowly exhale	❏	❏	_____
12.	Instruct patient to relax and breathe normally for a short time	❏	❏	_____

		S	U	Comments
13.	Instruct and encourage patient to gradually increase depth of respiration	❏	❏	_____
14.	Encourage patient to perform procedure 10 times every hour while awake	❏	❏	_____
15.	Offer mouthwash after spirometry is completed	❏	❏	_____
16.	Store spirometer in an appropriate place such as the bedside table until next scheduled time. Make certain spirometer is within easy reach of patient	❏	❏	_____
17.	Position patient as desired or ordered	❏	❏	_____
18.	Place call light within easy reach	❏	❏	_____
19.	Wash hands	❏	❏	_____
20.	Assess respiratory status and evaluate patient's response to spirometry	❏	❏	_____
21.	Document in nurse's notes: patient's respiratory status before and after incentive spirometry (the maximum of inspirations obtained in ml) and any adverse effects from the procedure	❏	❏	_____
22.	Do patient teaching	❏	❏	_____

Student Name _____ Date _____ Instructor's Name _____

PERFORMANCE CHECKLIST 2-3

TEACHING CONTROLLED COUGHING

		S	U	Comments
1.	Refer to medical record, care plan, or Kardex for special interventions	❑	❑	_____
2.	Obtain equipment	❑	❑	_____
3.	Wash hands	❑	❑	_____
4.	Don gloves	❑	❑	_____
5.	Introduce yourself	❑	❑	_____
6.	Identify patient	❑	❑	_____
7.	Explain procedure	❑	❑	_____
8.	Assist patient to upright position; place pillow between bed or chair and patient	❑	❑	_____
9.	Demonstrate coughing exercise for patient			
	a. Take several deep breaths	❑	❑	_____
	b. Inhale through nose	❑	❑	_____
	c. Exhale through mouth with pursed lips	❑	❑	_____
	d. Inhale deeply again and hold breath for a count of 3	❑	❑	_____
	e. Cough two or three consecutive times without inhaling between coughs	❑	❑	_____
10.	Abdominal or thoracic incision can be splinted before coughing with hands, pillow, towel, or rolled bath blanket	❑	❑	_____
11.	Encourage patient to practice coughing while splinting the incisional area once or twice an hour during waking hours; assist patient as indicated	❑	❑	_____
12.	Provide tissues and emesis basin for any mucus expectorated	❑	❑	_____

		S	U	Comments
13.	Provide washcloth and warm water for washing hands and face, provide mouthwash for oral hygiene, and return patient to comfortable position	❏	❏	_____
14.	Remove and dispose of soiled gloves and wash hands	❏	❏	_____
15.	Document exercises performed and patient's ability to perform them independently	❏	❏	_____
16.	Do patient teaching	❏	❏	_____

Student Name _____ Date _____ Instructor's Name _____

PERFORMANCE CHECKLIST 2-4

TEACHING POSTOPERATIVE BREATHING TECHNIQUES, TURNING, AND LEG EXERCISES

		S	U	Comments
1.	Refer to medical record, care plan, or Kardex for special interventions	❏	❏	_____
2.	Obtain equipment	❏	❏	_____
3.	Introduce yourself	❏	❏	_____
4.	Identify patient	❏	❏	_____
5.	Explain procedure to patient	❏	❏	_____
6.	Wash hands and don clean gloves	❏	❏	_____
7.	**Prepare patient for intervention**			
	a. Close door to room or pull curtain	❏	❏	_____
	b. Drape for procedure if necessary	❏	❏	_____
8.	Raise bed to comfortable working level	❏	❏	_____
9.	Premedicate with analgesic if indicated	❏	❏	_____

Postoperative Breathing Techniques

		S	U	Comments
10.	Place pillow between patient and bed or chair	❏	❏	_____
11.	Sit or stand facing patient	❏	❏	_____
12.	Demonstrate taking slow, deep breaths; avoid using shoulders and chest while inhaling; inhale through nose	❏	❏	_____
13.	Hold breath for a count of 3 and slowly exhale through pursed lips	❏	❏	_____
14.	Repeat exercise three to five times; have patient practice exercise	❏	❏	_____
15.	Instruct patient to take 10 slow, deep breaths every 1 hour until ambulatory	❏	❏	_____

	S	U	Comments

16. If there is an abdominal or chest incision, instruct patient to splint incisional area using pillow or bath blanket, if desired, during breathing exercises ❏ ❏ _____

Leg Exercises

17. Lifting one leg at a time and supporting joints, gently flex and extend leg 5 to 10 times ❏ ❏ _____

18. Repeat exercise with opposite extremity; lifting leg while supporting joints, gently flex and extend leg 5 to 10 times ❏ ❏ _____

19. Alternately point toes toward the chin and toward the foot of the bed four to five times ❏ ❏ _____

20. Make a circle with ankles of both feet four to five times to the left and four or five times to the right ❏ ❏ _____

21. Assess pulse, respiration, and blood pressure ❏ ❏ _____

Turning Exercises

22. Instruct patient to assume supine position to right side of bed; side rails on both sides of bed should be in up position ❏ ❏ _____

23. Instruct patient to place left hand over incisional area to splint it ❏ ❏ _____

24. Instruct patient to keep left leg straight and flex right knee up and over left leg ❏ ❏ _____

25. Place rolled bath blanket or pillow between legs ❏ ❏ _____

26. Instruct patient to turn every 2 hours while awake ❏ ❏ _____

27. Remove and dispose of soiled gloves and wash hands ❏ ❏ _____

28. Document and do patient teaching ❏ ❏ _____

PERFORMANCE CHECKLIST 2-5

APPLYING ANTIEMBOLISM STOCKINGS (TEDS)/SEQUENTIAL COMPRESSION DEVICES (SCD)

		S	U	Comments
1.	Refer to medical record, care plan, or Kardex for special interventions	❏	❏	_____
2.	Obtain equipment	❏	❏	_____
3.	Introduce yourself	❏	❏	_____
4.	Identify patient	❏	❏	_____
5.	Explain procedure	❏	❏	_____
6.	Wash hands and, if appropriate, don clean gloves	❏	❏	_____
7.	Prepare patient; close door to room, pull privacy curtain, and drape for procedure if necessary	❏	❏	_____
8.	Raise bed to comfortable working level	❏	❏	_____
9.	Examine legs and assess risk for conditions	❏	❏	_____
10.	Assess patient for calf pain or positive Homans' sign	❏	❏	_____
11.	Measure legs for stockings according to agency policy and order stockings	❏	❏	_____

Antiembolism Elastic Stockings

		S	U	Comments
12.	Assist patient to supine position to apply stockings before patient rises	❏	❏	_____
13.	Turn stockings inside out as far as heel; place thumbs inside foot part, and slip stocking on until heel is correctly aligned	❏	❏	_____
14.	Gather fabric and ease it over ankle and up the leg	❏	❏	_____

	S	U	Comments
15. Pull leg portion of stocking over foot and up as far as it will go, making certain that gusset lies over femoral artery; adjust stocking to fit evenly and smoothly with no wrinkles	❑	❑	_____
16. Repeat Steps 12 to 15 for opposite extremity	❑	❑	_____

Sequential Compression Devices (SCD)

	S	U	Comments
17. Place sleeve under patient's leg, with fuller portion at top of thigh. Some SCDs are knee-high	❑	❑	_____
18. Apply sleeve with opening at front of knee and closed portion behind knee. Some SCDs have a circular plastic inflatable sleeve	❑	❑	_____
19. When in place, make sure there are no wrinkles or creases in stockings; fold Velcro strips over to secure stockings, when appropriate	❑	❑	_____
20. Attach tubing to SCD after both sleeves are applied; align arrows for correct connection and appropriate effect; plug in and turn on unit	❑	❑	_____
21. Assess patient periodically	❑	❑	_____
22. Assess stocking at regular intervals	❑	❑	_____
23. Remove and dispose of soiled gloves and wash hands	❑	❑	_____
24. Document	❑	❑	_____
25. Do patient teaching	❑	❑	_____

Student Name _____ Date _____ Instructor's Name _____

PERFORMANCE CHECKLIST 4-1

CARE OF THE PATIENT IN A CAST

		S	U	Comments
1.	Patient teaching			
a.	Explain why the cast is being applied and how it will be applied	❑	❑	_____
b.	Advise the patient that the plaster cast will feel warm as it dries	❑	❑	_____
c.	Explain the extent of immobilization	❑	❑	_____
d.	Explain care of the cast and expectations after discharge	❑	❑	_____
e.	Instruct patient not to insert sharp objects (coat hangers or pencils) under the cast because these may abrade the skin and lead to infection	❑	❑	_____
2.	Handling the new cast			
a.	Support wet cast with the flat of the hands or on pillows	❑	❑	_____
b.	Place cotton blankets or other absorbent material under the cast	❑	❑	_____
c.	Expose the cast to air as much as possible	❑	❑	_____
d.	Turn the patient frequently to aid drying	❑	❑	_____
e.	Use a cast dryer or hair dryer on warm, not hot, setting to circulate air over cast	❑	❑	_____
f.	Do not apply paint, varnish, or shellac to the cast; plaster is a porous material that allows air to circulate to the skin	❑	❑	_____
3.	Skin care			
a.	Inspect skin at edges of cast and underlying cast for erythema and skin impairment	❑	❑	_____

			S	U	Comments
	b.	Remove plaster crumbs from skin with a washcloth moistened with warm water	❏	❏	_____
	c.	Use creams and lotions sparingly	❏	❏	_____
	d.	Apply waterproof material around perineal area	❏	❏	_____
	e.	Attend to patient's complaint to pain under the cast, particularly over bony prominences; if discomfort is not relieved by repositioning, report to physician; cast pressure may need to be relieved by windowing or bivalving	❏	❏	_____
4.		Turning to any position is generally permitted as long as the integrity of the cast is not compromised and the patient is comfortable; do not turn by grasping the abductor bar	❏	❏	_____
5.		Toileting—for a long leg or hip spica cast			
	a.	Use a fracture pan with blanket roll or padding as support under the small of the back	❏	❏	_____
	b.	Elevate the head of the bed, if permitted, or place the bed in reverse Trendelenburg's position	❏	❏	_____
6.		Abdominal discomfort			
	a.	Cast may be "windowed" (an opening cut into it) to provide relief of abdominal distention or a port for checking bladder distention	❏	❏	_____
7.		Mobilization			
	a.	Weight bearing is at the discretion of the physician, and the amount of weight bearing will be prescribed	❏	❏	_____
	b.	A cast shoe or a walking heel incorporated into a lower extremity cast will permit weight bearing without damaging the cast	❏	❏	_____

	S	U	Comments

8. Prevention of neurovascular problems (establish baseline measurements and assess neurovascular status before cast application; palpate distal pulses before cast application; assess color, temperature, and capillary refill of the appropriate fingers or toes; and assess neurological function, including sensation and motion in the affected and unaffected extremity)

   a. Perform neurovascular checks every hour for at least 24 hours after cast application; notify physician of color changes, alterations in sensation, or motion unrelieved by position change; cast may need to be bivalved (cut in two) to relieve pressure   ❏   ❏   _____

   b. Elevate affected extremity on pillows until danger of edema is over (usually 24 to 48 hours)   ❏   ❏   _____

   c. After mobilization of patient with lower extremity or upper extremity cast, avoid keeping extremity in dependent position for prolonged periods   ❏   ❏   _____

   d. After lower extremity cast is removed, encourage patient to wear elastic stocking and elevate affected leg at rest until full mobility is regained   ❏   ❏   _____

NOTES

NOTES

NOTES

NOTES

NOTES

NOTES

NOTES

NOTES

NOTES

NOTES

NOTES